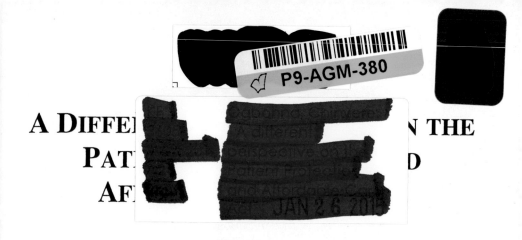

A DIFFE̶̶̶̶̶ N THE
PAT̶̶̶̶̶ D
AF̶̶̶̶̶

Chinyere Ogbonna

University Press of America,® Inc.
Lanham · Boulder · New York · Toronto · Plymouth, UK

Copyright © 2014 by
University Press of America,® Inc.
4501 Forbes Boulevard
Suite 200
Lanham, Maryland 20706
UPA Acquisitions Department (301) 459-3366

10 Thornbury Road
Plymouth PL6 7PP
United Kingdom

Library of Congress Control Number: 2013950512
ISBN: 978-0-7618-6184-3 (paperback : alk. paper)
eISBN: 978-0-7618-6185-0

Dedication

This book is dedicated to my wonderful students, who challenge me intellectually every day in class, with their incessant insightful questions, and to my amazingly wonderful and affectionate children, Nwachi, Chima and Chike McGruder, who challenge me to be the best that I can be as a mother, professor, and friend.

Dr. Ogbonna

Contents

Tables and Figures

Foreword

This book is timely and a valuable resource for understanding recent changes in the American health care system. It adds significance to the broader discourse on health care reform in the United States. Since President Lyndon Johnson signed the landmark Medicare and Medicaid laws of 1965, the U.S. health care system continues to evolve. All previous attempts for comprehensive health care reform failed until the United States Congress passed, and President Barack Obama signed into law the Patient Protection and Affordable Care Act or the Affordable Care Act (ACA) on March 23, 2010. The author argues persuasively that if this law is fully implemented the United States will move closer towards a comprehensive health care system. The ACA is designed to streamline health care delivery networks across the country, empower state governments to create their own marketplace that suits their local needs, improve quality, curb health costs, and expand access to more 30 million uninsured Americans.

This text enhances the reader's understanding of the evolution of health care reform in the United States and looks at the Affordable Care Act from a broader perspective. It first delves into a review of the various health care reform initiatives pursued at both the federal and state levels with emphasis on Tennessee's 1993 Medicaid reform known as TennCare, Oregon's 1989 Health Care Plan (OHP), and Massachusetts's 2006 Health Care Reform Plan. The state reform initiatives were driven by escalating Medicaid costs, decreasing state revenues and limited access to health care services by an increasing number of uninsured state residents.

The major emphasis of the rest of this volume examines the strengths, controversies, issues, and challenges of the Patient Protection and Affordable Health Care law. The message to the reader is compelling: the Patient Protection and Affordable Care Act is an important milestone in the slow and long road towards comprehensive health care reform in the United States. It is on course at transforming health insurance in the United States through collective responsibility. The current reforms of the insurance market reform means that discriminatory practices by insurance companies including exclusion of patients with pre-existing conditions ends, adding Americans ages 19 to 25 to their parent's plans is realized, and giving tax credits to needy individuals and families for purchasing insurance coverage is achieved.

In conclusion, Chinyere Ogbonna has written a readable text that is valuable to a broad spectrum of audiences including policymakers, professionals, health care analyst, and the general public. Students of health care administration and related fields will find that this book truly provides an in depth understanding of the evolving changes in the United States health care system.

Alex Sekwat
Professor and Associate Dean
Tennessee State University
January 2013

Preface

Research data show that Health care costs within United States were rising almost exponentially during the past few decades. These rising health care costs were cutting into state and federal expenditures, especially with the past recessions. As a result different States within the union tried various health care reform in their bid to curtail rising health care expenditures, especially expenditures relating to uninsured individuals. These health reforms were supposed to refigure the way that health care is provided for and paid for within their states. Amongst the most innovative State health care reforms were those carried out by the States of Oregon, Tennessee and Massachusetts. The basic tenets of the aforementioned state reforms were simultaneous expansion of health insurance to the previously uninsured or uninsurable and the curtailment of the states' rapidly rising health care costs.

Just like the different individual states, were experiencing fiscal strain from burgeoning health care costs, the Federal government's share of health care costs was also increasing drastically. Despite this increase in health care costs, there was no subsequent increase in the number of insured individuals. The uncompensated care received by uninsured individuals especially at Emergency rooms of hospitals was also a significant factor in the drastic increase of health care expenditures at both the state and federal government level. This state of affairs subsequently led to the enactment of the Patient Protection and Affordable Care Act (PPACA), which was signed into law on March 23, 2010, by President Barack Obama. The main objectives of the reform plan were to expand coverage and provide insurance for previously underinsured, uninsured and the uninsurable while at the same time trying to reduce health care costs by focusing on efficiency in the delivery of health care services. As such the law, specified Individual Mandate requirement, as a major component of the federal health reform law, as well as the provision of Essential benefits by insurance companies. The health reform law also paved the way for Health insurance exchanges where by individuals and small employees with less than 50 employees could buy health insurance. The bulk of the full aspects of the Affordable Care Act is not slated to go into effect until January 2014, but some of the preliminary portions of the Act that went into effect as of March 23, 2010 through late 2012, are discussed within this book.

This book describes the basic design, rationale, and anticipated benefits of the health care reform act as well as the challenges mounted by opposition to the health care act. The academic focus of the book is on a different perspective of the Affordable Care Act that would hopefully separate the rhetoric from the facts pertaining to the health care reform.

Since the reform has not yet been fully implemented in its entirety, this book is not geared towards the evaluation of the health care reform Act but upon presenting academic indicia relative to the health reform. This book is targeted towards Political science and Health care management/policy professionals and students, as well as individuals who are interested in learning more about the innovative Patient Protection and Affordable Care Act, (otherwise known as Obama care) that was enacted by President Barack Obama. Hopefully the book will proffer a different academic perspective to the Patient Protection and Affordable Care debate that is raging on in America today. May haps, generate interest in examining the law as a health policy initiative that can be tweaked to better fit the health care and health services needs of the nation and the goals of its enactment.

Acknowledgments

I appreciate the insightful comments and support Dr. Alex Sekwat, Associate Dean of Graduate Studies at Tennessee State University. I especially acknowledge the help provided by Andrew Doss, an undergraduate student at University of Tennessee, Knoxville, who was instrumental in helping with the formatting of the finished manuscript. I would also like to acknowledge my undergraduate public management, policy and criminal justice students at Austin Peay State University. They provided vocal support when I sometimes felt my academic intensity flagging during the process of completing this manuscript.

I extend my gratitude my three sons, Nwachi, Chima and Chike McGruder, and to the other myriad of individuals who cheered me on during this process.

Chinyere Ogbonna

Chapter 1

Introduction–Background Prior to Enactment of Patient Protection and Affordable Care Act

Health care is not just another Commodity. It is not a gift to be rationed based on ability to pay. It is time to make Universal health insurance a national priority, so that the basic right to health care can finally become a reality for every American. — Ted Kennedy former U.S. Senator [1]

Inherent in the idea behind the above quotation is that health care is a basic right, which should be available to every American. The health care system in United States is uniquely different from that of other nations, in that it is substantially more costly than any foreign system. In fact a 1998 OECD[2] health data report indicates that the health care system in United States is the most expensive, of all the industrialized nations, far outstripping the health care expenditures of any other country.[3] Studies also indicate that a large percentage of United States population was uninsured, more than any other industrialized nation.[4] These facts were the basis for the Patient Protection and Affordable care Act. The problem of increasing health care costs have led to different strategies, (both at the federal and different state levels) aimed at controlling growth of these health care costs, and finally culminated into the health reform act signed into law by President Obama on March 23, 2010. The law is known as the Patient Protection and Affordable Care Act (PPACA) or colloquially known as ObamaCare. In the past, the wide spread adoption of managed care with its austere and strict reimbursement rates and low national inflation rate, considerably slowed the rate of growth of medical spending. Despite this, a 1998 government study showed that health care expenditures would soon start increasing again, and there was the real possibility that it would double within the following decade,[5] if left unchecked or if nothing was done. It must be specified that the increased health care spending did not connote more insurance coverage for the uninsured or the uninsurable. Therefore it was obvious that tangible ways of keeping health care costs down were necessary so as to avoid the possibility of overwhelming the economy of the nation.

The issue of uninsured individuals had culminated in significant expenses and cost shifting. As of 2010, there were about 59 million uninsured Americans; the new health care reform law is projected to reduce the number of uninsured to about 23 million by the year 2019.[6]

Prior to implementation of PPACA, different states had enacted or were making moves towards the enactment of legislation that would reform the way health care was provided and paid for within their individual Medicaid programs. These actions were in response to rapidly escalating health care costs and uninsured care. This is due to the fact, that under a USA law, Emergency Medical Treatment and Active labor Act (EMTALA),despite being uninsured, individuals have to be stabilized if they had to go to the hospital for emergency care, regardless of their ability to pay or lack of insurance. This put the burden of uncompensated emergency room care on the hospitals, which then subsequently passed on the uncompensated care costs to other payers of healthcare. Prior to 1986, patient dumping or emergency care refusal were documented practices within hospitals with regards to dealing with uninsured patients or patients with the inability to pay, that present within emergency rooms at the hospitals. This practice was soon curtailed by the passage in 1986 of the Emergency Medical Treatment and Active labor Act (EMTALA), which mandated that all United States hospitals that receive Medicare Funds would have to evaluate and stabilize patients that present at Emergency rooms prior to releasing them.[7] It is important to note that EMTALA does not have a provision for reimbursement of the aforementioned mandated emergency medical services. The law is also applicable to all ambulance services within the United States thereby requiring bot hospitals and ambulance services to provide care to anyone that requires emergency treatment, regardless of the person's legal status, citizenship or ability to pay.

The passage of EMTALA, presented a social connotation with regards to health care and coverage discourse. The perception is that individuals without health Care insurance would not be left to die on the streets because hospitals are mandated to stabilize them if they present at the emergency room. As President Bush noted, "People have access to health care in America. After all, you just go to an emergency room." [8] But inherent in this ability to utilize hospital emergency room services, without the ability to pay, means that hospitals would be left with the cost of such uncompensated care. As such hospitals across the states within the nation were left with unpaid emergency medical bills as well as increasing expenses for care they provided to the uninsured. Thus the utilization of emergency rooms as a conduit for medical care and treatment for the uninsured and the uninsurable likewise had an effect on spiraling health care costs of states within the nation, especially considering the fact that it is a very inefficient mode of health care utilization. This is because hospital emergency room visits are disproportionately much more expensive than regular Health care provider office visits.

The State of Tennessee just like the other states within the nation was likewise battling high health care costs which were threatening to overwhelm the fiscal capabilities of the state. Thus on 1st January 1994, the state of Tennessee implemented a health reform plan for its Medicaid program known as TennCare. TennCare was implemented by the state of Tennessee in an effort to curb rapidly rising Medicaid health care costs while simultaneously providing greater coverage for previously uninsured patients. TennCare was one of the most bold and innovative health reform programs by a state to help curb its health care escalating costs. Continually escalating medical costs, growing uninsured populations with subsequent strained Medicaid budgets led different states such as Massachusetts, Maine, Oregon, Tennessee and Illinois to carve their own path in their efforts to reform their Medicaid plans within their individual states. These states crafted innovative reform programs to help cover the uninsured and curb their rapidly rising health care costs. This book will succinctly explore the basis for three of the most innovative State Medicaid health reform plans within United States as a basis or prelude to the Patient Protection and Affordable Care Act. The three unique and innovative health care reform plans undertaken by three different States of the union that are discussed within this book are TennCare, Oregon health plan and the Massachusetts reform health plan, but prior to discussing these three innovative state health care reform plans, it is important to first of all comprehend how health insurance process works within USA.

Overview of How Health Insurance Worked Prior to Enactment of Patient Protection and Affordable Care Act

The health insurance process is a system whereby a large pool or group of individuals or in some instances just single individuals pays a monthly premium to buy into a specific health insurance plan. This health insurance plan will cover the cost of stipulated medical expenses as delineated by the plan. There are usually copayments, coinsurance and deductibles, out of pocket Maximums, maximum allowable benefits and coverage exclusions by the insurance.

Copayment or Copay is a fixed fee each member must pay upon receipt of heath care; the insurance company pays the balance. The copays for specific services are specified up front by the insurance plans and are usually printed on the front of the health insurance card. Thus an insured person is cognizant of the fact that every time to go to see a doctor or health service provider, they would have to pay a copayment. The copayment is supposed to deter insured individuals from over utilizing the services of doctors or health care providers. Thus the idea is that it would hopefully preclude insured individuals from going to a health care provider every time they have a minor ailment or the sniffles. The copayment would thus be the impetus that would deter insured individuals from utilizing the services of a health care provided except when truly needed. In practice, the copay actually saves health insurance companies millions of dollars in unnecessary health care visits. For instance let's assume an insured individual goes to a gynecologist for irregular menstruation. If the insurance plan of the insured female stipulates $40 copay for specialist visit (the gynecologist is considered a specialist), that is the amount she would pay and the balance of the cost of her gynecological visit will be billed to her insurance company.

Co-insurance is different from copay in that coinsurance, applies once the deductible has been met, but before the out of pocket maximum has been reached. Once the deductible has been met, then the insured individual is responsible for coinsurance if applicable until the out of Pocket maximum has been reached. With coinsurance, the actual amount paid by the insured is dependent on the cost of health care services provided. Thus if the health plan has a 90/10 coinsurance, then for instance if the cost for a problem oriented gynecological exam is $1000 and that particular patient's coinsurance is 10% then that particular patient would have to pay $100 which is 10% of the cost of the gynecological exam. Therefore, with coinsurance the fiscal burden on the insured is more if the cost of services rendered are higher and vice versa. With Copay the amount paid by the patient is the same regardless of the cost of services rendered for that particular health care provider visit.

The deductible is the fixed out of pocket amount the insured would have to pay usually for each insured year, prior to the insurance company covering most if not all of the insured's major medical costs for that particular year. Such major medical costs would include hospitalization and surgery costs. But just about all health insurance plans allow individuals to use some services, like emergency room or routine doctor's annual checkups, without first meeting the deductible. For such visits the stipulated copay applies. Since the copay is not subject to the deductible, i.e. you can utilize your copay without first meeting your deductible for medical visits, the dollar amount paid for co-pay is not applicable towards your deductible. Since deductibles are annual, they are reset at the end of each year. Depending on the insurance company, once an insured individual has reached their deductible for that year, they would still have to pay their copay since the copay is not applicable towards the deductible, and they are only finically responsible for, their monthly premiums and coinsurance if applicable during the duration of the rest of the year. The health insurance plan would specify the deductible for both single and for family. The deductible for family is usually close to double the deductible for single insured individuals. The higher the deductible the less the monthly premiums, thus some individuals might chose a plan with higher deductible but lower premiums if they are healthy and do not foresee utilizing a lot of health care for that particular year. If one is chronically ill and utilizes a lot of health care services then it would make sense to choose a plan with low deductible and higher monthly premiums.

The Out of Pocket maximum is the stipulated amount by the health insurance plan that an individual has to spend for their covered medical expenses before the plan can pay for 100% of medical expenses for the plan year, usually with the exception of copayments. Copayments are usually required by most insurance companies, regardless of if the deductible and the out of pocket maximum have been met. It is important to remember that monthly premiums and copayments do not add towards, out of pocket maximum, only the deductible and the coinsurance apply or add up to the out of pocket maximum. Thus once an individual have reached their maximum out of pocket payment for the year, they do not have to pay any more coinsurance for the rest of the year. The concept of the out of pocket maximum protects the insured in the instance of catastrophic medical occurrence and subsequent expenses.

Exclusions refer to what the Health insurance plan would not cover, for instance most health insurance plans would not cover the cost of cosmetic procedures like botulinum toxin (Botox) injections to prevent wrinkles, or breast augmentation, except if those procedures have specific medical benefits.

Lifetime Maximum benefits refer to the most that the health insurance plan would pay for medical benefits, including medications, over the course of a lifetime of an insured individual. That means that once the insurance company had paid a total of the dollar amount specified within its lifetime benefits for that particular individual , it is not obligated to pay a cent more towards the cost of provision of health care for that particular individual. Different health insurance plans have varying lifetime maximums. The lifetime maximum can range from $40,000 to $4 million to unlimited or no lifetime limit. Of course the best insurance plan for most individuals would be one without a lifetime limit, because the cost of health care services has been rising exponentially over the past 2 decades, so much so that the cost of a patient being hospitalized for a stroke can run in the hundreds of thousands of dollars, for just one stroke incidence and hospitalization and the cost of caring for an individual with Spina Bifida can run to over $2 million.

Thus, for instance, John Doe, an insured individual has a lifetime maximum benefit of $1 million, and he has had several heart attacks which required several hospitalizations and treatments. The costs of his hospitalizations and treatments totaled about $1milllion dollars, he was informed by his insurance company that he has reached his life time maximum limit and as such the insurance company is not obligated to pay any more money towards the costs of his medical expenses. A few days later during John Doe's routine colonoscopy , it was found that he had a couple of polyps in his colon that were pre metastasized, but his insurance company would not cover cost of removal of the polyps, nor cost of the colonoscopy, since he had reached his life time limit. If John could not afford the cost of the surgery, he would not have the polyps removed which would eventually metastasize and cause his death. So prior to enactment of the Patient Protection and Affordable Care Act, it was imperative that individuals be cognizant of their particular health insurance life time limits.

Therefore, under the concept of health insurance, the cost of care for members of a pool or group of individuals is spread over the whole group. The members of that insurance plan pay a premium. Some of the premiums are utilized in the payment of healthcare services of sick members of the plan. As such Health insurance works on the premise that within members of a health insurance pool or plan, the healthier members subsidize the cost of treatment of the sicker members of that particular health insurance plan. Thus a plan with a lot of healthy individuals that pay their premiums month after month for years will work very well, whereas a health insurance plan with lots of sick members that will require costly medical treatment will not be fiscally solvent, regardless of whether plan members pay their monthly premiums steadily over the years.

Invariably health insurance plans serve the purpose of providing a means of access to care, since with health insurance one can go visit their medical providers for needed medical services. Research indicates that people with health insurance have better access to care, especially since they are more likely to have a regular doctor. [9]

There are various individual, private and public health insurance plans or coverages. Medicaid and Medicare are examples of public health insurance. Other public insurance programs cover Federal and State Government employees, Native Americans, veterans, members of the military, low-income children, and others.[10] Then there is private insurance, the majority of private health insurance is provided by employers, through employer sponsored group health plans. With regards to an employer sponsored health plan, the employer covers a large portion of the employee's monthly health insurance premiums and a smaller portion of applicable family members' portion within the health plan, as part of the benefits provided to the employee in lieu of higher pay. These insurance benefits are not regarded as income and as such the employees with such benefits are not taxed on the monetary value of the portion of the health insurance benefits paid for them by their employers. A small employer with less than 50 employees may buy health insurance through a small group market whereas a large employer with more than 50 employees may buy health insurance through a large group market.

Then there are some individuals that buy their health insurance plans through the individual insurance market. They have to buy their health insurance through the individual market, otherwise known as residual market, because they are not eligible for group health plans or they do not qualify for government or public health insurance programs like Medicaid and Medicare. Within the individual market, the health plan may cover the individual as well as applicable family members, but in this instance the individual purchaser, pays all the premium costs.

Table 1.1- Source of Health Insurance Coverage for Persons the Age of 65 or Younger* in 2010 [11]

Employer	156.5 million people	58.9%
Medicaid	44.1 million people	16.6%
Medicare	7.3 million people	2.8%
Individual	16.8 million people	6.3%
Uninsured	49.9 million people	18.8%

*Excludes individuals in the armed forces.

As can be seen from the table above, if an individual can't get private or government (public) or individual insurance then they may go uninsured.

It is important to note that prior to enactment of Patient Protection and Affordable care Act, about 50 million non-elderly Americans were uninsured. Accordingly "Most of the uninsured have low incomes, below 200 percent of the federal poverty level (or $44,700 for a family of four). Most of the uninsured are full-time workers and their family members, whose jobs don't offer health benefits.

This is a changing group of people; many people who are uninsured one year are insured the following. And millions of people who have insurance today may be counted among next year's uninsured. An estimated 32 percent of Americans and their families had a gap in health insurance for at least one month, and 87 million people were uninsured at some point during 2007 and 2008."[12]

Some individuals can also be underinsured meaning that their insurance plans will not cover their catastrophic health services costs nor provide adequate access to care. Lack of adequate access to care can occur if the individual's insurance plan does not reimburse the health care provider a fair rate. When that occurs, some providers will shirk from accepting as patients insured individuals from such plans, with the result that there would be a dearth of health care providers who will accept that individual's health care plan for compensation for health care services provided. This fact can also lead to great financial distress for those that are underinsured should they happen to get catastrophically sick.

From the later part of the 1970's, most health insurance models usually followed the indemnity plan otherwise better known as the fee for service. This is a health insurance plan, whereby the insured individual has complete autonomy in choosing the health care provider to utilize; the insurance company will pay for the services of the health care provided minus the deductible and coinsurance where applicable. This type of insurance is the least restrictive of all the available insurance plans.

Then there is the Health Maintenance Organizations (HMO). HMOs are managed care plans that have lower monthly premiums than the other health insurance plans but these plans are the most restrictive of all the health care plans. The HMO pays a fixed monthly fee or capitated fee per enrollee per month to the physician or health care provider based on the number of HMO enrollees that choose that provider as their primary care physician. So for example if there are three hundred insured individuals of a specific HMO that have Dr. A , as their primary care physician, and assuming the HMO paid $8 capitated payment per patient per month to Dr. A. Therefore, Dr. A would receive $2400 per month capitation from that particular HMO for those three hundred patients, regardless of if the patients utilize the services of Dr. A that month or not. Conversely, if some of the 300 patients require medical services for that particular month that costs more than the $2400 provided the doctor by the HMO, the doctor would not be getting any more extra money from the HMO for that particular month. Thus there are some financial risks involved for a doctor that has a capitated agreement with an HMO for a specific number of patients. So, with this type of insurance plan, it makes sense for the health care provider to minimize the utilization of health care services by the insured each month, because regardless of the amount of utilization by each enrollee per month, the health care provider is still paid a set specific amount per each enrollee per month.

The main focus of health maintenance organization is on preventive care. With this type of insurance plan, the insured would have to choose a primary care provider within network (that is a part of the HMO Plan), who will be the point of contact between the insured and other specialists if and when necessary. It is important to note that with the HMO plan, the insured can only utilize the services of the health care providers, i.e. doctors; hospitals, clinics etc. within the HMO plan or network, and can only see a specialist upon the referral of the primary care provider or physician. If the insured chooses to utilize the health care services of a specialist without the referral of the primary care physician (who acts as a sort of gatekeeper to other doctors or health care specialists that are affiliated with the HMO), the HMO would not pay for such utilization of services. A lot of insured individuals who have HMO insurance have them because that is the only insurance their employers provide or because they are generally cheaper than the other insurance plans or types.

Preferred Provider Organization (PPO) health plan is a plan whereby the health insurance has negotiated low reimbursement rate for health care services with different Health Care Providers, Doctors, Nurses, and Clinics. Under this plan, the insured still has the option of going outside the providers that have the arrangement with the insurance plan, but the insured cost sharing will be much lower within the preferred provider network than utilizing health care services of providers outside the network. This fact encourages insured individuals within the PPO to try to utilize health care services of providers within network, so as not to pay the higher health care costs associated with going out of network for health care services. For instance if a Woman decides to have tubal ligation done within network, the insurance might cover 90% of her costs within network, but only 70% of her costs out of network and in addition she may also be responsible for the difference between what the surgeon charged and what her PPO plan had negotiated with the surgeon as customary pay for such tubal ligation. PPO is closest to fee for service, because under PPO, a doctor or provider is paid for each service rendered albeit an agreed discounted payment.

Then there are Point of Service (POS) Insurance plans. These are offshoots of the HMO, but with more control by the insured. Under this type of Health insurance plan, the insured has 3 points of Services it can utilize for the provision of needed Health care services.

1) The insured can utilize the health care services of a Primary care Physician as per under HMO guidelines whereby the physician is supposed to make the determination regarding referrals and specialist needs.
2) The Insured can receive their health care services through a Preferred provider organization (PPO) under the PPO in network rules,
3) The insured can receive needed health care services outside of the HMO or PPO networks, within out of Network rules of the plan, which usually indicates that the insured pay a higher copay or coinsurance when utilizing out of network services.[13]

Thus within the Point of Service plan an insured person can utilize health care providers outside the insurance health plan, though doing so would be more expensive and complicated for the insured, since the insured would have more out of pocket expenses.

A fifth health insurance plan is the Exclusive Provider Organization (EPO) plan which is a bit similar to the HMO plans in that enrollees need a primary health care provider gatekeeper or doctor that would refer them to specialists as well. This type of health insurance plan is likewise also focused on preventive care and they encourage enrollees to engage in behavior that will have positive benefits on their health. Enrollees have to pay a copay when they visit their primary care doctor, similar to HMO's and other health plans. And like HMO's they do not cover health care services provided by non-network health care providers. But unlike HMO's, they do not offer capitated payments to their health care providers, instead they pay doctors and other health care providers a discounted fee based on health care services provided. The EPO is quite restrictive, in fact it is more restrictive than HMO's because they do not have the range of doctors or providers within the plan as do HMO's while at the same time they do not cover services rendered by doctors or providers that are outside their network. So it can sometimes be difficult for an insured individual to find a specialist within the specific EPO that they want, but the advantage of this health care plan is that it is generally cheaper than the HMO.

Thus the above health care plans are examples of health care plans that individuals can choose from within USA. It must be noted that indemnity health insurance plans are no longer as prevalent as they were back in the later part of the 70's and through the early 2000. But invariably health plans offer some sort of assuredness to policy holders that they would be covered in the unfortunate event that they get sick, though the degree and depth of coverage depends on the specific health insurance plan and specific individual policy.

---

1. Kennedy, E. M. (2003). Quality, Affordable Health Care for All Americans. American Journal of Public Health, Volume 93(1), 14.
2. OECD stands for Organization for Economic Cooperation and Development.
3. A Comparative Analysis of 29 Countries. (1998). OECD Health Data. Paris: Organization for Economic Cooperation and Development
4. Ibid
5. Smith, S., Freeland, M., Heffler, S., McKusick, D., & Health Expenditures Projection Team. (1998). The Next Ten Years of Health Spending: What Does the Future Hold? Health Affairs 17, no. 5, 128-140.
6. Foster, R. (2010, April 22). Estimated Financial Effect of the Patient Protection and Affordable Care Act. Retrieved August 2, 2012, from CMS:https://www.cms.gov/ Research-Statistics-Data-andSystems/Research/ActuarialStudies/downloads/ PPACA_2010-04-22.pdf
7. Stevens, R. (2007, September 21). History & Health Policy in the United States: Putting the Past Back. Retrieved August 7, 2012, from Investigator Awards: http://www.investigatorawards.org/downloads/research_in_profiles_iss21_sep2007.pdf
8. Ibid
9. Why Do You Need Health Insurance? (n.d.). Retrieved Januray 7, 2013, from Agency ForHealthCareReasearchandQuality:http://archive.ahrq.gov/consumer/insuranceqa/insura nceqa3.htm
10. A Health Insurance Overview. (n.d.). Retrieved January 2, 2013, from Health Insurance 101: The Basics: http://101.communitycatalyst.org/basics/overview
11. Ibid
12. Ibid
13. Health Insurance Explained. (n.d.). Retrieved January 4, 2013, from Insurelane: http://www.insurelane.com/health/health-insurance-explained.html

Chapter 2

Basis for TennCare Implementation

During the late 1980s and early 1990s, a majority of the states in United States were in the middle of a health care crisis exacerbated by recession and rising health care costs. In the light of this situation many states implemented various health care reforms. By mid 1990s, eight states had enacted laws that were geared toward the goal of ensuring access to medical care for all of their citizens.[1] Up till then, except for Hawaii, none of the states that had previously enacted universal coverage laws since 1993 had fully implemented them.[2] These states were not able to do so because of a federal law, namely the Employee Retirement Income Security act (ERISA) of 1974, which barred states from requiring employers to offer health benefits. In order to require employers to provide health insurance coverage for their employees, a state would have to win a congressional exemption from ERISA.[3] Hawaii was the only such state to be granted such an exemption because its Prepaid Health Care Act was passed before ERISA became law. Apart from the obstacle posed by ERISA, any attempt to achieve universal coverage and tighter cost control must be coordinated with the Medicare program.

By early 1990s, the states were being encouraged to try new ways of financing and delivering health or medical care. This was shown by willingness of the federal government to waive Medicaid requirements that prevented innovation by states. Tennessee took advantage of this option.

Like most of the other states, Tennessee faced major health care system problems. Medicaid spending and the number of enrollees in the state within the Medicaid program, had grown so rapidly in past years[4] that health costs for enrollees, were starting to threaten financial stability of the state's treasury. At the beginning of 1993, several years of burgeoning growth in Tennessee Medicaid expenditures had created a budget crisis that affected the entire state government.[5] The increase in the number of eligible Medicaid recipients as well as health care cost inflation had nearly tripled health care expenditures in just five years. Just like in so many other states, Medicaid spending was the second largest and fastest growing item in Tennessee's budget.[6] In fact cost of the program had grown so steeply and rapidly, that it threatened the viability of all other functions of Tennessee state government. Out of all the states in the union, Tennessee was ranked 11th in terms of Medicaid enrollee numbers and was 17th in total Medicaid expenditures.[7] This was despite the fact that an estimated 470,000 Tennesseans were without health insurance. Medicaid growth had exceeded the ability of the state to sustain through normal methods of state revenue generation.[8] The state could no longer afford the uncontrollable expansion in Medicaid program costs, so a better solution had to be found.

In Tennessee, as with other states in United States, the largest portion of health care expenditures goes to the hospitals. Total Medicaid costs in Tennessee grew from approximately $692 million in fiscal year (FY) 1988-1989 to almost $2.7 billion in FY 1993-1994, while number of Medicaid recipients increased from 540,000 to almost 1 million. The compounded average annual growth in number of enrollees was 13.1%, and the average cost per enrollee increased at a rate of 7.4% per year.[9] Despite the fact that Tennessee had a high Medicaid eligibility standard,[10] as mentioned previously, it ranked 11th when compared with other states in terms of Medicaid enrollees and ranked 17th in total Medicaid expenditures.[11] Tennessee also ranked 44th nationally in per capita income, but relative amount of money spent on hospital care in Tennessee increased when measured as a percent of total state per capita income. In 1973, Tennessee was ranked 4th in United States, but by 1981, the state's rate of increase had risen, whereby Tennessee was number 1 in the country with regards to Medicaid hospital care expenditures, per percentage of Tennessee per capita income.[12]

Conversely, the increasing health costs incurred by the state were not resulting in increased quality of care or adequate access to care.[13] In addition a lot of needy people such as the working poor and the uninsured were excluded totally from public health assistance under Medicaid with no other available health insurance option. Although about 70 % of the uninsured had jobs or were dependents of employed persons, medical benefits were usually not offered at their jobs, and their wages were generally too low to pay for high premiums usually charged insured people that were not part of a large employee group. Therefore it would seem more beneficial to these workers to lose their jobs so as to be qualified for Medicaid thus discouraging indigent individuals from taking employment due to fear of losing their Medicaid benefits.[14]

In view of the problems faced by Tennessee, the then Governor, Ned McWherter, upon assuming office had managed to keep costs down by utilizing "creative financing" techniques. These techniques included provider taxes repaid through Disproportionate-Share Hospital (DSH) payments and other enhanced provider payments. These tactics were used to induce hospitals and nursing homes to fund some of the state's share of Medicaid Costs. This practice was fundamental in bringing about an increase in federal medical assistance percentage from 67.6 to about 83.1 percent during initial years of McWherter's administration, while simultaneously keeping Tennessee's medical spending costs down. The state thus had managed to hold down increase in its general revenue fund appropriations for Medicaid to less than 25 percent, despite the fact that the program's budget increased threefold during this period.[15]

The State was able to keep its costs that low, during this period, because of its maneuvering of the Disproportionate-Share Hospital (DSH) payments. Under federal law, when determining payment rates for inpatient hospital care, state Medicaid programs are required to "take into account the situation of hospitals that serve a disproportionate number of low income patients with special needs." This requirement is known as the Medicaid disproportionate share hospital (DSH) payment adjustment.[16] The Boren Amendment as established in (OBRA) Omnibus Budget Reconciliation Acts of 1980 and 1981 was legislation that brought into place the DSH program. This piece of legislation tried to maintain access to health care for all, by mandating that states should consider special payment needs for hospitals that serve a large portion of Medicaid and uninsured patients. The reason was that hospitals that render high volumes of care to low income individuals usually lose money due to low Medicaid reimbursement rates.[17] These hospitals were also losing money because they generally provided high volumes of care to indigent patients and therefore had high levels of un-compensated care. Usually such hospitals with large caseloads of low-income patients generally have low private caseloads, thus making it harder for the hospitals to shift cost of uncompensated care to privately insured patients.[18]

The DSH payment legislation was enacted in the early 1980s but the different states did not really pick up on benefits of utilizing it, till beginning of 1990s. Disproportionate-Share Hospital expenditures soared in the 1990s and by 1996, they accounted for one out of every eleven dollars spent on Medicaid.[19] By early 1993, new federal laws designed to curb utilization of "creative financing" techniques were being implemented.

The most important of these laws was the 1991 federal law known as Medicaid Voluntary Contribution and Provider Specific Tax Amendments of 1991 (P.L. 101-234).[20] The body of this law has requirements that would virtually eliminate provider donations as well as restrict provider taxes. As such, the 1991 law contained several restrictions for money that would be eligible for federal matching funds, thus making provider donations technically impossible, while at the same time bringing about a restriction in provider taxes. The federal Medicaid requirements were also changed so as to eliminate federal match for voluntary provider donations. The law was directly related to flagrant abuse of DSH payments and as such it was intended to regulate the way that states generated funds that would be utilized for attracting matching federal Medicaid funding.[21] Key provisions of the law included:

1) Banning provider donations;
2) Limitation of provider taxes so that provider tax revenues could not exceed 25 percent of each individual state's share of Medicaid expenditures;
3) Imposition of provider tax criteria so that taxes were "broad based" and providers were not "held harmless,"[22]

4)   Capping DSH payments at about 1992 levels.[23]

The restrictions brought about by enactment of the 1991 law may be summarized as follows: Health care-related taxes that are eligible for federal matching funds must be broad-based, imposed uniformly and include all members of a class, such as all inpatient hospitals, all physicians or all HMOs and prepaid entities; taxes cannot make up more than 25 percent of a state's share of Medicaid; and taxes cannot also contain a "hold harmless" provision, which guarantees that health care providers will have the tax that they paid returned to them.[24]

It was difficult for states to establish tax and donation programs that complied with the 1991 law. Thus this law subsequently curtailed DSH payment growth and forced many states to restructure DSH financing and look for other ways of keeping their medical budget in balance.[25]

Prior to enactment of the 1991 law, utilization of "Creative financing" techniques by different states was possible simply because in 1985, Health Care Financing Administration (HCFA), started allowing states to include voluntary provider donations in calculation of federal matching payments under Medicaid. This made it possible for any individual state to collect voluntary provider donations to fund its Medicaid program. In Tennessee, this donation would be matched by the federal government at slightly better than two to one. These tactics were utilized to induce hospitals and nursing homes to fund part of the state's share of Medicaid costs, since they would receive higher Medicaid reimbursements in return.[26] Around 1980s, some states began to adopt provider tax programs, which operated along the same lines as the voluntary provider donation programs. These programs were of great financial benefit for the states that utilized them.[27] Each dollar of revenue raised from either a tax or donation program, could bring in one to four federal financial participation (FFP) dollars depending on the state's federal matching rate.[28] The following is an example of how a Medicaid DSH program worked prior to the 1991 Law:

1)   The state receives $20 million from a provider, in donation or tax.
2)   Since DSH payments are match able Medicaid expenses, the federal government can reimburse the state anywhere from 50 to 80 percent of the DSH payment, depending on the state's federal matching rate. Assuming the rate for this state is 50 percent, the federal government would then reimburse the state half of the $20 million and that would be $10 million.
3)   The state then makes a DSH payment back to the provider as a lump sum payment or as an increase in Medicaid reimbursement rate. In this case the state makes a $22 million DSH payment to the same provider that made the donation of $20 million. Thus the provider has earned $2 million in DSH payments while the state is short $2 million of the matching federal fund of $10 million.
4)   The deal is concluded with the provider receiving $2 million extra in DSH payments, while the state had received $8 million (i.e. $10 million

minus $2 million, it had to pay for DSH), in federal money without having to spend any of its own funds. The federal government has thus paid $10 million in DSH payments, whereas only $2 million of it was paid to DSH provider, while the state kept the balance.[29]

Such tactics were responsible for overwhelming growth in Medicaid DSH payment/utilization, and subsequent percentage increase of federal medical assistance from 67.6% to about 83.1%. Therefore it was possible for different states to control individual increases in their respective general fund appropriations for Medicaid, despite almost a threefold increase in general Medicaid budget. The Medicaid DSH payments thus made it possible to spend tax and donation revenues, especially since DSH payments were not subjected to the Medicare upper payment limit. So states could make practically unlimited DSH payments while earning FFP dollars in the process.[30]

Starting from Oct. 1, 1992, a state's disproportionate-share payment[31] could not exceed 12 percent of its total Medicaid budget, but states above that limit could continue at their current percentage, while states below that limit could not surpass 12 percent. Thus enactment of this law made it mandatory for more than 30 states that had engaged in this type of funding to change the way that their Medicaid programs were funded.[32] This law thus curbed as well as changed the way that states could generate funds to attract matching Medicaid federal dollars.

Due to restrictions of the 1991 law, states then turned to intergovernmental transfer[33] (IGT) programs as their primary revenue source for their DSH programs.[34] Under these programs states would transfer funds from public institutions such as state psychiatric facilities, university hospitals and county and metropolitan hospitals to state Medicaid agency. The state would then make DSH payment back to these facilities while collecting federal matching Medicaid dollars in the process.[35] Since the IGT mechanism was billed as DSH payments to public facilities, it had the added advantage (over provider tax and donation programs) of preserving federal dollars for local and state institutions.[36] But, depending on the specifics of a program, private hospitals could be completely excluded under an IGT-financed DSH program.[37]

Implementation of the 1991 law curtailed DSH spending growth, but emergence of these IGT programs were of concern to federal policy makers. Policy makers questioned the appropriateness of DSH payments in certain circumstances, and they were especially concerned that some states were making DSH payments to facilities that were not large Medicaid providers.[38] Policy makers were also concerned that some other states utilized DSH payments which over compensated providers for unreimbursed costs incurred in caring for Medicaid and indigent patients. Thus some providers were getting DSH payments that exceeded the revenue that they received for rendering care to Medicaid patients.[39] In a nutshell, federal policy makers did not believe that DSH payments were being utilized for the intended purpose of helping safety-net providers.

Instead they believed that DSH payments were being used to help general state financing.

In fact a 1993 survey of 39 states utilizing DSH programs indicated that 33 percent of their DSH funds were retained by the states rather than being paid to disproportionate-share hospitals.[40]

To address these issues, Congress included the following provisions to OBRA in 1993:

1)   In order for a hospital to receive DSH payments, it should have a Medicaid use rate of at least 1 percent.

2)   A single hospital could not receive total DSH payments that exceeded the unreimbursed costs of providing inpatient care to Medicaid and uninsured (charity care) patients. These limits were effective in 1994 for most public hospitals and in 1995 for private hospitals.[41]

The provisions contained in the 1991 and 1993 laws, were critical in spurring different states to explore different avenues of managing their Medicaid programs, since they could no longer depend on DSH payment windfall. Thus during that period, several of the states enacted or were in the process of enacting reforms in the way that their Medicaid or public health care insurance programs are administered. As of January 1995, ten states had gotten waivers from Health Care Financing Administration (HCFA),[42] to reform the administration of their health care programs especially Medicaid. These states included Arizona, Florida, Hawaii, Kentucky, Ohio, Oregon, Rhode Island, South Carolina and Tennessee. Six other states also had waiver submissions with HCFA. These six states included Delaware, Illinois, Louisiana, Massachusetts, Missouri and New Hampshire. Ten other states were considering waiver submissions, and these states included California, Connecticut, Kansas, Maryland, Nevada, New Jersey, New York, Oklahoma, Texas and Washington.[43] These states hoped to achieve autonomy in the way that they managed their Medicaid programs. They were hoping that this autonomy would be utilized in developing cost-sharing provisions or cost reduction techniques, such as shifting of Medicaid enrollees from a fee for service system to that of a managed care system.[44] This shift would supposedly result in savings to states that chose to undertake this route. Therefore this shift had the most impact on states that have tried to reform their Medicaid programs.[45]

After implementation of the 1991 and 1993 laws, Tennessee was faced with the possibility of losing $494 million in federal matching funding. Governor McWherter had to act so as to circumvent the crisis that could result from loss of matching federal funding.[46] The state could not afford to wait for a national health system reform to address the financial and access problems posed by Medicaid.[47] It was then necessary to formulate a different policy that would take into account problems facing the state with regards to increasing Medicaid costs and uninsured population.

These specific problems faced by Tennessee in managing its health care had to be taken into account when structuring a reform program or plan. Drastic reductions in coverage did not seem like a feasible solution since a large number of Tennessee's indigent population were already not insured under Medicaid.[48] So it was necessary to consider fundamental reform of the Medicaid program.

According to McWherter (1993), the state of Tennessee considered three policy options and they were as follows:

1) Substantial annual tax increase: This was not a fiscally or politically tenable option as Tennessee had not been a very wealthy state. Moreover Tennessee's constitution prohibits a state income tax. The state had tried to raise health care funds by levying a 6.7% broad-based tax on hospitals and other professional services. But health care organizations vigorously opposed this idea and the federal government restricted this method for increasing federal contributions to state Medicaid programs. The resultant decrease in federal funds made the state's financial crisis worse.

2) Massive reduction in reimbursement rates and in provision of healthcare services: This would also be impractical as these reductions would not solve the ultimate problem of high health costs. It would instead encourage cost shifting to insured or private pay patients, while at the same time reducing access of Medicaid recipients to health care services. This process would also shift the site of these services from preventive or ambulatory clinics to more expensive hospital outpatient departments or emergency departments. And since these were indigent patients they would still be unable to pay for the cost of their hospital emergency room visits.

3) Fundamental health care reform: This seemed to be Tennessee's only realistic option and this would include major reform of both health care delivery system and financing system.[49]

On April 8, 1993, the then democratic governor of Tennessee, Governor Ned McWherter announced the broad outline of TennCare program. The overall general goals of the program being the following: Global budgeting, Standard benefit package, Pooling of purchasing power, Managed care, Incentives for preventive care, Elimination of inappropriate welfare benefits, Cost sharing, Quality control, and the elimination of class distinctions.

TennCare would hopefully assure cost neutrality for the federal government and also reduce health care costs for all levels of government from what they would have been under the Medicaid system. Former Governor Ned McWherter believed that TennCare would expand coverage to virtually every uninsured person in the state without reduction of services or increase in taxes. Instead this goal would be achieved by utilizing proposed cost savings that would be gotten from managing Medicaid as a managed care program. Implementation of TennCare needed approval from Health Care Financing Administration (HCFA) and waiving of key regulations governing Medicaid programs. Governor Ned McWherter submitted TennCare proposal to HCFA as a section 1115 research and demonstration waiver request on June 16, 1993.

On November 18, 1993 after protracted negotiations involving White House and Department of Health and Human Services (DHHS), the Clinton Administration granted Tennessee a waiver that would allow it to provide health insurance for 1.5 million poor and uninsured people. Under TennCare proposal the state would shift 1 million Medicaid recipients into private managed care plans that would compete for patients across 12 regions of the state.[50]

The state of Tennessee has seen three governors take office since TennCare was implemented. The state is currently under the governorship of Governor Haslam, who succeeded Governor Bredesen as the Governor of Tennessee. Governor Bredesen and his predecessor Governor Sundquist cumulatively instituted many sweeping changes to TennCare program in an effort to cut the rising cost of the program. The majority of the changes started in 2000, when the reform program started to unravel. There were continuing problems with management of the program, high turnover of TennCare managerial positions as well as problems with Blue Cross of Tennessee. At the same time medical providers became increasingly reluctant to accept new TennCare patients, especially since the payments for services rendered were not guaranteed. The problems escalated, such that by the beginning of 2002, TennCare was consuming about 26% of the state's budget. As such the growing consensus was that the program should be scaled back. When the Section 1115 waiver was renewed in 2002, the federal government backed out of contributing to the cost of expansion of coverage. As a result of the waiver, financial eligibility levels were lowered for TennCare. This meant that income levels needed to qualify for TennCare insurance were decreased substantially. Therefore individuals that previously qualified for TennCare were now considered to be earning too much money to be eligible for TennCare. Thus, thousands of prior premium paying people were systematically dropped from TennCare rolls, because they earned much more money than was eligible for inclusion into TennCare. There was also implementation of a redetermination process that was user unfriendly resulting in the dis-enrollment of individuals who were actually eligible for TennCare. The state has also instituted major reductions or elimination of coverage for citizens with chronic diseases.

Governor Bredesen announced on January, 2005, that part and parcel of his TennCare reform plan would result in the termination of coverage for adults on TennCare Standard[51] and TennCare Spend Down. By the first week of June, 2005, about 200, 000 adults that were on TennCare Standard had received letters notifying them that they were no longer eligible for TennCare standard but they should submit application for TennCare Medicaid. Termination letters for TennCare Spend down enrollees were slated to be sent out towards the later part of June 2005.[52]

According to TennCare Information, as of 2006, TennCare would no longer cover the following:

- Adults who were previously covered as uninsurable or medically eligible;
- Adults that have Medicare but do not receive Supplemental Security Income (SSI);
- Adults that were previously covered because they had catastrophic medical bills and thus were able to qualify for Medicaid Spend Down (Medicaid Spend Down or Medically Needy coverage allows people with catastrophically high medical bills to get on TennCare. Prior to April, 29, 2005, people older than 65, the blind, the disabled and single parents were considered, but as of 2006 only children and pregnant women are considered).[53]

As of 2006, the following were still eligible for TennCare Medicaid coverage:

- Children under 21;
- Pregnant women;
- Families that were on Families First;[54]
- Individuals that receive SSI check;
- Women currently on treatment for breast or cervical cancer;
- Individuals that live in nursing homes with a monthly income that is below $1,373, or receives long-term care services that are paid for by TennCare;
- Individuals who stopped receiving SSI since November 13, 1987, while still living in Tennessee;
- Individuals who had previously received SSI and Social Security Check together at least once in the same month since April, 1977 and who still currently received Social Security Check.[55]

There were still continuing changes to TennCare prior to enactment of the Patient Protection and Affordable Care Act. Some of the TennCare changes included, increased focus on quality. In 2006 TennCare began to require that their managed care network acquire National Committee on Quality Assurance (NCQA) accreditation.[56] Also during that same year, the state mandated TennCare MCO's to report their HEDIS measures.[57]

Thus far the HEDIS 2010 results showed that there was a general improvement in 6 out of 8 adult diabetes measures from 2006 to 2010. There were also improvements in 5 out of 6 women's health measures from 2006 to 2010, children's health measures improved 12 out of 12 during the same period, and 10 out of the 12 children's health measures exceeded national Medicaid average for 2010.[58]

Under the recent Affordable Care Act, there are certain mandatory requirements that will affect TennCare. Some of the recently implemented ones include the smoking cessation coverage for pregnant women as well as changes in home health criteria that require a doctor visit prior to getting a prescription. There are likewise planned future requirement under the auspices of the new Act. Some of the most notable ones include the requirement to increase primary care provider payments to 100% of Medicare by January 1, 2013. Also there is the requirement that all individuals under age 65 who are not eligible for coverage under Medicare and who have incomes below 138% poverty level be covered by TennCare.[59]

The Oregon Health Plan (OHP)

Another state that had to reform its Medicaid program was Oregon. Oregon's Medicaid health care reform was one of the most controversial. The Medicaid health reform plan enacted by the State of Oregon is known as the Oregon Health Plan. Dr. John Kitzhaber, initially spearheaded the efforts for the plan, initially as a State Legislator and then later on as the Governor of the State of Oregon. Dr. John Kitzhaber was formerly an emergency room physician prior to joining the state legislature. Starting from 1989, Oregon initiated a series of health reform plans with the end goal of attaining universal coverage. The health reform plans included a mandate for employers to provide health coverage for their employees.[60] The employer mandate did not go into effect, thus the focus of the health reform plan was on Medicaid expansion of OHP. The plan likewise utilized state certified insurance packages for small businesses and the self-employed as well as a high risk medical insurance pool.[61] But the crux of the Oregon health plan was the intent to expand coverage to previously uninsured while at the same time reducing the scope of health services covered. Thus the plan would cover greater number of poor or indigent Oregonians, which are individuals with incomes below 100 percent of the federal poverty level, while simultaneously limiting the scope of health benefits and services provided. Therefore such individuals would be offered a basic health benefit coverage that would be more limited in scope than traditional Medicaid.[62] As such, the plan worked in principle based on a prioritized list. The list ranked health care conditions and treatments based on clinical effectiveness and cost-effectiveness. The plan would then cover health conditions that could be effectively and efficiently treated, but the plan likewise emphasized prevention and patient education.[63] It also tried to control costs while improving access by enrolling Medicaid recipients in capitated managed care organizations. Capitated managed care organizations are structured to control medical costs by limiting utilization, as such each health care provider, has a built in incentive to minimize the scope and rate of utilization of health care by individual patients. The plan was predicated on ranking treatments that helped prevent disease, higher than services that treated diseases after they occurred. As such, it would be more likely to cover procedures that prevented diseases than procedures that simply sought to treat the diseases after their onset.

The OHP would then provide coverage for treatments that were ranked on a covered Prioritized List line for the client's reported medical condition.[64] Every couple of years, the Oregon state legislature would draw a line on the list of possible health care services, and Oregon Medicaid would pay for all health services above the line and would not pay for any of the health services below the line. For instance the OHP would not cover certain transplants. That was true of such transplants that were very expensive and had been deemed of minimal increment to length of life or with minimal increase in length of life. The thinking was that the money recouped thus by rationing care would be utilized elsewhere where the medical services would provide appreciable health care benefit. Thus in 1989, the state legislature enacted a schema that would essentially end expensive coverage of services that would have been provided expensive care to only a limited number of beneficiaries. Such costly health care services were regarded of limited benefits, and the presumption was that the savings would be shifted to more cost effective services for existing and new Medicaid enrollees, thus expanding coverage while at the same time keeping costs down. Prior to making the determination with regards to services that would be covered, the State formed an eleven member Health services Commission. Oregon Health Decisions sponsored eleven public hearings, forty-seven town meetings, and to better learn about the values and preferences of the citizens regarding their thoughts about prioritizing medical situations, commissioned a telephone survey.[65] Based on all the information gathered thus, the commission compiled a list of medical procedures and compared the procedures to Quality of Well-Being Scale. The scale measured indicia of health wellbeing after treatment or utilization of needed medical procedures.

Thus Oregon would measure the Quality of Wellbeing scale against the cost of health services and their attendant contribution to length and quality of life. Based on those parameters, the commission then listed about 1,600 medical procedures in order of priority on a "Cost/Utility Ratios Report."[66] There was a lot of attendant controversy concerning the mechanism of the report, so much so that the commission decided to redo the process again. They released a new rank ordered list on February, 20, 1991. This list had about 800 items and the actuary had attached cost coefficients to each individual item. Legally the legislature could not rearrange items on the list; they simply had to consider their State's fiscal prerogatives and then draw a line through the list demarcating what would be covered and what would not be covered. Procedures above the line would be covered under the State's Medicaid program whereas procedures below the line would not be covered under Medicaid.[67]

The savings from the elimination of coverage for less effective procedures as well as the managed care programs were intended to fiscally allow the State to expand their Medicaid eligibility level from 58 percent of the poverty level to 100 percent of the poverty level. This would provide Medicaid coverage for about 118,000 more indigent Oregonians. This idea utilizes the utilitarian principle of providing the greatest good for the greatest number of people, whereby public funds would be utilized to promote the greatest good for the most people.

Simultaneously, Oregon had also passed two mandates. One of the mandates, required employers that did not have health insurance coverage for their employees, to either provide the newly defined benefits package or pay additional payroll taxes. The other mandate required coverage for the uninsurable by the creation of an insurance pool.[68] The idea was that the employee mandate, the creation of the insurance pool as well as the efficient coverage utilizing the cost/utility ratios would help the state achieve almost universal coverage of its uninsured and uninsurable population. Since Medicaid is a federal law, there were some stipulations to what could be covered and essentially the state of Oregon would be eliminating some basic Medicaid health services. Oregon had to get approval from Health Care Financing Administration in the form of an administrative waiver under the demonstration authority of Section 1115 of the Social Security Act. It is important to note that Medicaid was brought into play as a Title XIX program of the social Security Act of July 30, 1965 [69]

Just like Tennessee did with implementation of TennCare, Oregon had to get a federal waiver in order to implement the health reform plan as a Section 1115 Medicaid demonstration project. But the State's initial waiver application in 1989 was not approved until 1993, and that was mainly due to the fact that the plan triggered a national debate about health care rationing.[70]

But rationing of health care is already part and parcel of the United States health care system. The high cost of medical and preventive care, in most instances can lead to non-utilization of preventive care or lack of early treatment of health conditions, and this neglect sometimes resulted in delayed and more expensive treatment for non-insured patients,[71] which they could likewise not afford to pay. This lack or non-utilization of preventive care by uninsured people can be considered a sort of rationing. Rationing of healthcare is a process whereby, access to Health care is limited or curtailed as a result of certain factors. Such factors can include price, ability to pay, and insurance. For instance, individuals without health care insurance can choose to self-ration their health by not going to the doctor for health care services if they are sick, simply because they cannot afford the cost of such provider services. Or a health insurance plan may choose to ration care by not covering certain services, for instance a health insurance plan might decide not to cover noninvasive (Magnetic Resonance Imaging) MRI-guided focused ultrasound ablation for uterine fibroids, simply because of the cost of such a procedure and the fact that it is a new and innovative procedure.

For instance Harvard Professor Michael Katz and Princeton Professor, Harvey Rosen, defined rationing as such:

> Prices *ration* scarce resources. If bread were free, a huge quantity of it would be demanded. Because the resources used to produce bread are scarce, the actual amount of bread has to be *rationed* among its potential users. Not everyone can have all the bread that they could possibly want. The bread must be *rationed* somehow; the price system accomplishes this in the following way: Eve-

ryone who is willing to pay the equilibrium price gets the good, and everyone who does not, does not.[72]

Inherent in the above explanation is that individuals have to ration, because supplies are not unlimited and resources are not unlimited. This counters the perception of the public that private industries do not ration especially private insurance companies. But they do, when an insurance company decides they do not cover certain services, either because they are experimental and the costs of the particular health care services are prohibitive, or because the benefits of those particular health care services are not apparent or effective, they are in reality, rationing the provision of certain health care services. This is also the case if a particular insurance company decides to have a 40% coinsurance on the exorbitant price of biologic specific drugs. They are effectively putting that drug out of the price range of a lot of their beneficiaries that need it. But most, of the critics of the PPACA, do not consider that particular brand of private insurance rationing as such. Instead they consider the private health insurance companies as prudent and efficient private industry managers, that are providing beneficiaries a choice or discretion to choose to pay the coinsurance and buy the drug or not to, regardless of the fact that the coinsurance makes it out of the reach of the specific beneficiaries.[73] But conversely if the government were to refuse to cover certain procedures because the insurance managers of that particular health pool do not consider such procedures efficient and effective use of taxpayers' money, most critics would contend that, that was unjustified rationing of health care on the part of the government.[74]

Author Uwe Reinhardt, writing for the New York Times, put the perspective on rationing, based on his research literature and media reports of our health care system, succinctly as such:

- Many Americans without health insurance or very high deductibles routinely forgo[75] prescribed medicine or follow-up visits with a doctor because they cannot afford it, risking more serious illness later on.
- A 2008 peer-reviewed study[76] by researchers at the Urban Institute found that health spending for uninsured nonelderly Americans is only about 43 percent of health spending for similar, privately insured Americans. Unless one argues that the extra 57 percent received by insured Americans is all waste, these data imply rationing by price and ability to pay.
- A few years ago, The Wall Street Journal featured a series of articles reporting how often uninsured middle-class Americans are charged the highest prices at pharmacies and in hospitals, and how sometimes they are hounded over medical bills to the point of being jailed for failed court appearances.
- Studies have shown that solid middle-class American families — even ostensibly insured families — can lose all of their savings and some-

times their homes[77] over mounting medical bills in the case of severe illness.

- In its report Hidden Cost, Value Lost: The Uninsured in America[78], the prestigious Institute of Medicine a few years ago estimated that some 18,000 Americans yearly die prematurely for want of the timely health care that health insurance makes possible and that can prevent catastrophic illness.
- A recent study by an M.I.T. professor found that uninsured victims of severe traffic accidents receive 20 percent less health care than equivalent, insured victims and are 37 percent more likely to die from their injuries[79].

According to Dr. Arthur Kellermann, professor of emergency medicine and associate dean for health policy at Emory University School of Medicine, in a National Public Radio interview, "In America, we strictly ration health care. We've done it for years."[80] Accordingly he stated the following: "But in contrast to other wealthy countries, we don't ration medical care on the basis of need or anticipated benefit. In this country, we mainly ration on the ability to pay. And that is especially evident when you examine the plight of the uninsured in the United States."[81]

He went on to recount the following incident that occurred with regards to a young mother of two that was admitted more than 15 years ago to his emergency room after suffering a hemorrhagic stroke. "We worked for 90 minutes to save her life, but basically she had burst a blood vessel in her head. She didn't have a chance." "She had no health insurance, and when the money got tight, she had to make a choice — she could either buy the groceries for her kids, or she was going to buy the three blood pressure medicines she had to take every day."[82] Dr. Kellermann went on to further elaborate that, "for less than the cost of that futile, 90-minute effort in the ER, the woman could have had all the blood pressure medication she needed for the rest of her life. It was not a government bureaucrat who decided she should forgo treatment until it was too late — it was her own lack of health insurance that led her to make that choice."[83] In this instance the rationing was patient led rationing, the woman did not have the resources to pay for both her groceries and her medications so she decided to ration her medication in lieu of not buying groceries with catastrophic result in this particular case.

Regardless of whom doles out the rationing, the fact is that health care rationing is part and parcel of health care provision within United States, the national and media focus on the rationing inherent within the Oregon Health plan was intense. There were various critics both in academia and from affected interest groups, who criticized both the general approach and the original list. These critics raised objections within and outside the state.[84] But the reasoning inherent in the idea of the health plan was the notion that it was not feasible for everyone within the state to get all the medical care that they would need or want. So the underlying premise was that any coverage was better to have for the about 400,000 Oregonians that did not have private health insurance nor qualified for Medicaid.[85] The snag was that such universal access would come at the opportunity cost of limited health services to those on Medicaid rather than the standard coverage available on private health insurance. Neither the government nor the private sector could tenably afford unlimited health services to everyone, and as such the State had to demarcate the adequate minimum level of health coverage.[86]

The reasoning did not deter the magnitude of criticism. The extent of the criticism prompted the health Services Commission to go back and redo the process all over again taking into considerations some of the critic's objections. After some changes, the state resubmitted its waiver request and it was finally granted the federal waiver in 1993, albeit later than expected for their health reform plan. Initial studies of Oregon health plan's early performance from 1994-1998 were for the most part favorable. The first year of the plan's operation in 1994, saw an increase of about 120,000 new enrolled members. Likewise bad debts at Portland hospitals from uninsured patients dropped about 16%. The state was able to extend new Medicaid coverage to more than 100,000 eligible beneficiaries, thereby reducing the uninsured rate in 1992 from 18 percent to 11 percent by 1996.[87] The state likewise initially mitigated critics' fears of the plan's rationing impact on Medicaid patients by minimizing extensive rationing and offering generous benefit packages. For instance the initial earlier version of the bill had precluded reimbursement reduction without subsequent corresponding reduction in provision of required services. In 1990, that language was changed to indicate that the state, as determined by an independent actuary, would pay rates that were necessary to cover the cost of services provided.[88] That appeared very generous and fair to providers that were especially cognizant of Medicaid low reimbursement policies within other states. It was also important that the enrolling of beneficiaries in managed care plans proceeded smoothly, because of these initial encouraging signs a bipartisan political coalition supported the OHP and thus protected it from initial budget battles. The referendum to raise cigarette taxes to fund the health care plan was twice approved by voters.[89]

The health plan had undergone some changes since its inception especially during the 2001–2003 period when the state had one of the highest unemployment rates (7.4 percent) in the nation.[90] This was crucial to some of the subsequent problems of the health plan because the state of Oregon was dependent to a large extent on personal income tax. The health plan had seen its budget increase from $1.33 billion in 1993-1995 to $2.36 billion in 1999-2001, and with the high unemployment rate in the state as well as the state's fiscal tightness, it was important to try and rein in the costs. It was also during this period that the state decided to apply for a new waiver to expand the health plan.

Oregon state officials submitted a request in 2002, for a federal waiver to amend their demonstration project by creating Oregon Health plan two (OHP2), which would be an expansion of the original Oregon Health Plan. The federal waiver was submitted through the then new Health Insurance Flexibility and Accountability (HIFA), initiative. The expansion would increase the plan by about 46, 000 enrollees, and this would be carried out by raising OHP's Medicaid eligibility level from 100 percent to 185 of the federal poverty level over a period of time.[91] The hope was to gain federal matching funds for the previously state funded Family Health Insurance Assistance Program (FHIAP), which would help enable its expansion. [92] The waiver was granted in October 15, 2002, during one of the highest unemployment rates of the state, but that fact did not deter the state from moving forward with its expansion efforts.

Since state funds were limited, OHP2 had to provide fewer services for more people; benefits were reduced for covered enrollees, such that the state could generate more funds to bring in more uninsured Oregonians into the health plan. The state also wanted to finance the increased coverage by the division of the health plan into two components the OHP Plus and OHP Standard.[93] The populations that were specifically eligible for Medicaid would be covered by OHP Plus with benefits based on the prioritized list. Such populations would include children and pregnant women[94] that earned up to 185% of the federal poverty level. On the other hand, in a move guaranteed to enable the state receive additional federal matching funds for the expansion population; Oregon meshed its Family Health Insurance Assistance Program (FHIAP), which previously subsidized private health insurance premiums for low-income individuals, into OHP Standard.[95] The expansion population which included couples, single adults and parents that were not eligible for Medicaid under federal guidelines would receive reduced benefit package that was about 78 percent of OHP plus value and be covered by the new OHP Standard instead. But OHP standard enrollees would still have their covered services ranked according to the prioritized list, but they would likewise have new copayments ranging from a $5 for a doctor's visit to a $250 per hospital admission copayment. Also the OHP standard enrollees would not receive dental, mental health, vision services and nonemergency transportation.[96] Prior OHP copayments had been minimal and rare. OHP standard enrollees would also have increased premiums, with tightened enrollment rules and providers, i.e. physicians and Pharmacists would have the option not to provide services for OHP standard beneficiaries that could not pay their copayments. At this point, OHP Standard began to enforce strict premium payment policies, including having enrollees wait six months before they could re-enroll into the program if they miss a premium payment.[97] The plan closed further enrollment into OHP, in August of 2004, and placed more limits on hospital services. Beneficiaries that did not pay their premiums were permanently dropped from the program and not allowed to re-enroll.[98]

Because of Oregon's fiscal straits, the state requested a federal permission waiver to have an enrollment cap for OHP Standard, which would allow it to either decline new enrollees or set lower poverty level eligibility standard, depending on availability of state funds. The waiver also allowed the state, the power to possibly reduce, if necessary, the benefit package of OHP standard to the actuarial equivalent of federally mandated Medicaid minimum, without having to go through further approval from the Centers for Medicare and Medicaid Services (CMS).[99] It was important for Oregon to have this authority so as to be able to decrease the covered services on their prioritized list, without having to go through CMS, each time they needed to do so. The hope of the policy makers was that this waiver would provide the state with the needed flexibility and tools to limit OHP spending.[100]

The changes were supported by bipartisan legislature in Oregon, because of the fiscal constraints of the state, since it appeared that the new cost-sharing and premium policies were the only feasible option for coverage expansion as well as reduction of the state's uninsured population.[101]

As a result of all these restrictions to the Oregon Health Plan, and reduction of benefits, the number of eligible residents covered by OHP Standard dropped dramatically. About 88,874 residents were enrolled in the plan as of March 2003, but by September 2003, enrollment had decreased to about 50,000, and by October of 2004, enrollment in OHO Standard had further decreased to 46,520 and the Oregon Association of Hospitals and Health Systems were reporting in November of 2004, that charity care at the state's hospitals had doubled since the cuts.[102] The state of Oregon, reintroduced some of the previously eliminated OHP standard benefits in summer of 2004, and in response to a lawsuit and subsequent court ruling, ended the recently introduced OHP Standard copayments for adult enrollees.[103] Nonetheless by early 2005, the number of enrollees in OHP Standard had dropped to 38,000, and the Department of Human Services announced that enrollment would have to drop to 24,000 for the program to remain financially solvent. The department also briefly considered the possibility of eliminating the $6 premium for people making less than $770 per month, but then decided against the idea, since that would have been too expensive for the state to forgo such premiums. The state continued to have plummeting enrollment, by late 2007, enrollment was at 19,000 and by early 2008 it was at 18,000, bringing the number of uninsured Oregonians to 615,000, which was about 17 percent of the population.[104]

Because of the rapidly decreasing enrollee rolls, OHP Standard announced in January 2008, that it would accept new enrollees for the first time since 2004. This move would allow new members to make up or take the place of members that had disenrolled.[105] Subsequently, Oregon's State Department of Human Services announced that it would utilize a lottery process to enroll 3,000 new members in March, and another 3,000 new members in April. More than 83,000 uninsured Oregonians entered their names into the lottery.[106]

John Kitzhaber took office again for a third term as governor of Oregon in January 2011. Since taking office he has proposed new reforms and cuts to OHP plus, in order to help reduce escalating Medicaid costs within his state. For the period 2011-13, the state faced an $860 million gap between funding and costs for nearly 600,000 people on the Oregon Health Plan.[107] The Governor had proposed to reduce the gap by trimming $570 million from administrative costs and health plan benefits as well as a 19 percent reduction in Medicaid payments to doctors and other providers for health services rendered. The remaining $290 million shortfall, he wanted to cover through health care reform.[108] To that end, Coordinated Care Organizations (CCOs) were created within the state to help reduce spiraling health care costs by streamlining preventive care and treatment and preventing inefficiencies within the system. Thus over two legislative sessions encompassing the period 2011 through 20012, Governor Kitzhaber and bipartisan lawmakers passed the legislation for CCOs.

The CCOs are health plans that consist of various health care providers, who have agreed to work and collaborate together within their community in delivery of streamlined health care services for Oregon health plan enrollees.[109] Enrollee's medical benefits will remain the same under CCOs, but in lieu of separating physical, behavioral and other types of care, which is very inefficient and costly; these Care organizations would better coordinate services and focus more on prevention, chronic illness management and person-centered care. They would likewise have the flexibility within their budgets to provide services alongside the current OHP medical benefits with the goal of meeting Triple Aims of better health, better care and lower costs for the population they serve.[110] These Coordinated Care Organizations are local and they are allotted one budget that would grow at a fixed rate that would be utilized for the provision of physical, mental, and dental care. Such care organizations are responsible for the health outcomes of the enrollee population that they serve; as such there is an inherent partnership between healthcare providers, community members and health system stakeholders that have financial responsibility and attendant risks.[111] The CCOs started in some Oregon communities in August of 2012, and as other CCOs are formed, they would enroll OHP beneficiaries between September 1 and November 1, 2012.[112] Therefore most Oregon Health Plan members would have access to coordinated care by September 1, 2012.

Preliminary third party analysis indicated that the State of Oregon could save significant projected short and long term costs by the utilization of CCOs. State and federal projected saving by the analysis, would be more than $1billion within 3 years and more than $3.1 billion over the next five years.[113] It would be interesting to see how Oregon would integrate it health reform with the new mandates of the Patient Protection and Affordable care Act, but the expansion mandate of the PPACA might feasibly mesh in seamlessly with the bold reform that is known as the Oregon Health Care Plan.

Massachusetts Health Care Reform Plan

On April 12, 2006, under the governorship of Mitt Romney, the State of Massachusetts signed legislation that would provide nearly universal health care coverage to state residents. The bipartisan legislation combined the concept of individual responsibility through the requirement of an individual mandate on the purchase of health insurance with government subsidies to low income individuals so as to ensure affordability. The individual mandate simply meant that citizens of the state were required to have health insurance otherwise they would face a penalty, unless if they fell within specific exceptions. Implementation of

the plan began at the end of 2006. By May 2007, over 100,000 previously uninsured people had gained coverage. Full implementation of the reform act was
expected by July 1, 2007. The goal of then Governor Romney, in signing the
legislation was to provide "every citizen with affordable, comprehensive health
insurance."[114] Therefore the Massachusetts health Reform law mandated that
every resident of the state should have health insurance coverage, regardless of
if it were from the government or the private sector, otherwise they would have
to pay a tax penalty. Residents of the state without Minimum creditable coverage would be assessed monthly penalties that were cumulative for the months
without affordable health insurance, and were due at yearly tax filing times; they
would also lose their $219 income tax personal exemption.[115] Likewise there
were tax penalties on employers that failed to offer or provide health insurance
plans for their employees.

The penalties assessed to citizens were half the cost of the lowest-priced
Commonwealth Choice plan available to the individual, and they varied by age
or income based on percentages of the Federal Poverty Guidelines (FPG). So
individuals that their incomes were at or below 150% of the FPG did not have to
pay an uninsured penalty.[116]

Table 2.1- 2012 Tax Year Penalties

Income and Age	150.1- 200% FPG	200.1- 250% FPG	250.1- 300% FPG	Above 300% FPG Age 18-26	Above 300% FPG Age 27+
Tax Penal- ty	$19 per month $228 per year	$38 per month $456 per year	$58 per month $696 per year	$83 per month $996 per year	$105 per month $1260 per year

Source: MassResources.org. 2012.[117]

Individuals within the state with limited incomes may be eligible for
MassHealth or Commonwealth Care, which were state run health insurance. In
order to meet the general requirements so as to be eligible for MassHealth, the
individual must live in Massachusetts, have low to medium income and must be
within one or more of the following categories:

- a family living with children under the age of 19 years
- a pregnant woman with or without children

- a person who is long-term unemployed
- a disabled person
- an adult who is working for a qualified Employer[118]
- a person who is HIV positive
- a child under the age of 19 years
- an adult Caretaker relative[119] living with children under 19 years of age when neither parent is living in the home
- elderly (65 or older)
- a woman with breast or cervical cancer
- a person in need of long term Care[120]
- a young adult under age 21 who was in the care and custody of the Department of Children and families (DCF/DSS) on his/her 18th birthday.[121]

All other residents within the state were mandated to buy health insurance if "affordable" insurance was available.[122] Under the reform law, the state government would provide a regulated minimum level of health insurance coverage as well as the provision of free health insurance for residents that earned less than 150% of the federal Poverty level. The focus of the health care law was on providing coverage within a three year period for the majority of the state's 500,000 uninsured population.

The Health law of 2006 also created an independent public Commonwealth Health Insurance Connector Authority or the Health Connector. The functions of the health connector included acting as an insurance broker that offered private insurance plans to residents. It also helped the residents and businesses of Massachusetts find and pay for health insurance[123] that was within their means. The Health Connector ran Commonwealth Care which was funded by the state. Commonwealth Care was a program that provided health insurance for low and moderate-income Massachusetts residents who otherwise did not have health insurance. Commonwealth Care enrollees or beneficiaries got free or low cost health services through different managed care health plans. The beneficiaries could choose from any of the managed care plans depending on their need and level of income. The health managed care plans were offered by private insurance companies and there were variations in cost of plans,[124] depending on income limits. For instance the income limit for the state for 2012 is listed below. An individual may be eligible for Commonwealth Care if their family's annual income was at or below 300% of the Federal Poverty Level (FPL).

Table 2.2- Family Size for Income at or below 300% FPL[125]

Family Size	Income at or Below
1	$33,516
2	$45,396
3	$57,276
4	$69,156
5	$81,036
6	$92,916
7	$104,796
8	$116,676

Although a resident had to have a gross income no more than 300% of the federal Poverty guideline, (FPG) to be eligible for Commonwealth Care, there were still different plans for different income limits within that indication. According to MassResources.org, the following income limits were applicable to different plans.

- If your income is 100% FPG or less, you do not have to pay monthly premiums.
- If your income is 150% FPG or less, you do not have to pay monthly premiums if you choose the lowest cost plan offered in your area. If you choose a higher cost plan, you will have to pay a monthly premium.
- If your income is more than 150% FPG but not more than 300% FPG, you must pay monthly premiums that depend on income, where you live, and the plan you choose.
- Everyone must pay copayments for prescription drugs.[126]

Table 2.3- Commonwealth Care Cost Summary by Plan Type

	Plan Type 1	Plan Type 2		Plan Type 3	
% FPG	0-100%	100.1-150%	150.1-200%	200.1-250%	250.1-300%
Monthly Premium (for lowest cost plan)	$0	$0	$40	$78	$118
Preventive Services	$0	$0		$0	
Office Services (PCP/Specialty)	$0	$10/ $18		$15/ $22	

Radiology (X-Ray, Lab Work)	$0	$0	$0
Imaging (MRI, CAT, PET)	$0	$30	$60
Outpatient Surgery	$0	$50	$125
Emergency Room Visits (no copay if admitted)	$0	$50	$100
Hospital Stays (Inpatient)	$0	$50	$250
Prescription Drugs: Generic Preferred Not Preferred	$1*/ $3.65 $3.65 $3.65	$10 $20 $40	$12.50 $25 $50
Contraception Prescriptions	$0	$0	$0
Mental Health/ Substance Abuse (Outpatient, Inpatient, Methadone)	$0/$0/$0	$10/$50/$0	$15/$250/$0
Vision (Exam, Glasses)	$0/$0	$10/$0	$20/$0
Max Out-of-Pocket (Medical/Pharmacy)	$0/$250	$500/$750	$800/$1500

Source: MassResources.org[127]

Thus the tables above clearly indicate that if an individual qualified for Plan type 1, there was no monthly premium payment, but for individuals that qualified for plan type 1 but chose plan type 2A, they had the option of selecting a health plan with a zero premium or they may choose to select a health plan other than the $0 premium plan, in which case the individual would have the responsibility of paying the monthly premium for such selected plan. On the other hand, Members within Plan Type 2B and 3 must pay monthly premiums, though these premiums were based on income and selected health plan.[128]

Table 2.4- Copay Information by Plan Type

Plan Type 1	The copays for pharmacy services for both first-time prescriptions and refills are: • $1 for generic drugs and over-the-counter drugs • $3.65 for brand-name drugs There is a $250 copayment maximum for pharmacy services during a benefit year. Your benefit year is from July 1- June 30 each year. Once you have been charged $250 in pharmacy copayments during a benefit year, you will no longer pay copayments for pharmacy services until the next benefit year. You may apply for a **copayment wavier** for up to twelve months if you believe you have experienced extreme financial hardship affecting your ability to pay. Only certain events are considered extreme financial hardship. Contact Member Service if you want to learn more about applying for a copayment waiver.
Plan Type 2A	Plan Type 2A members are responsible for copays. View the **Health Benefits and Copays** chart for copay cost. If you are enrolled in a $0.00 health plan you may apply for a **copayment waiver** for up to twelve months if you believe you have experienced extreme financial hardship affecting your ability to pay. Only certain events are considered extreme financial hardship. Contact Member Service if you want to learn more about applying for a copayment wavier.
Plan Type 2B and Plan Type 3	Plan Type 2B and Plan Type 3 members are responsible for copays. View the **Health Benefits and Copays** chart for copay cost. Plan Type 2 members have a $500 copayment maximum for pharmacy services during a benefit year. There is a $750 copayment maximum for all covered services excluding prescriptions. Plan Type 3 members have an $800 copayment maximum for pharmacy services during a benefit year. There is a $1250 copayment maximum for all covered services excluding prescriptions. Your benefit year is from July 1- June 30 each year. Once you have been charged the maximum in copayments during that benefit year, you will no longer have to pay copayments for that type of service until the next benefit year.

If you change your health plan and want the copayments you have already paid under your old plan to count toward your maximum copays for your benefit year, you must ask your old health plan for a Copayment Transfer Letter. Your old health plan will send you this letter and you will need to give this letter to your new health plan. The letter will tell your new health plan the amount of copayments already paid during the year. You must send this Copayment Transfer Letter to your new health plan within 45 days from when your coverage begins in your new health plan or you may not be able to adjust your maximum copays for your benefit year. If you have any questions about this process, contact the health plan that you are currently enrolled in.

Source: Health Connector, Commonwealth Care Program Guide[129]

There are other general stipulations needed to be eligible for Commonwealth care insurance. The general criteria are below for residents of the state:

- You are age 19 or older
- You are uninsured; or you are paying full premium costs (e.g. under COBRA); or you are in a waiting period for coverage
- You cannot get coverage as a dependent on a family member's group plan
- You are not eligible for MassHealth, TriCare, the Insurance Partnership, the Unemployment Medical Security Program, the Fishing Partnership Health Plan, or mandated SHIP college student insurance
- You meet the income limits
- You are a citizen or eligible noncitizen
- Your current employer (or a family member's employer) has not offered you group health insurance in the past six months where:
  o the employer covered at least 20% of the annual premiums for the family plan
  o and 33% of the annual premiums for the individual plan[130]

Generally, Commonwealth Care was for adults, whereas children could be covered under MassHealth in lieu of Commonwealth Care.

Despite the fact that the cost of health care as well as the yearly rate of increase was still a challenge in MA, studies showed that to the extent that the State of Massachusetts sought to decrease the number of uninsured citizen, the Massachusetts health reform plan was successful. The health insurance reform of the state was effective in significantly increasing the number of insured within the state from about 90 percent insured to about 98 percent insured, which was the highest percent of insured within any state in the nation,[131] and Massachusetts had about 99.8 percent of all the children within the state insured.[132] The national average for uninsured adults during that period was about 16 percent. So the health care reform process added about 401,000 more to the insured category. Out of those numbers, 79% or 318,000 of the lately insured were due to public health insurance programs, 154,000 were enrolled at Common wealth Care, 83,000 purchased individual insurance and 164,000 were enrolled in MassHealth. But it is still, important to note that private or employer sponsored health coverage was the dominant source of health insurance coverage within the state, covering about 79 percent of the insured. That is pretty impressive. The state was able to implement all this while maintaining public support for the insurance reform. According to Blue cross foundation report, as of 2011, about two thirds of adult residents of Massachusetts approved of the health reform plan, and the majority of employers within the state believed that the health reform effort had been good, for the state. Interestingly about 88 percent of Physicians in Massachusetts thought that the reform efforts either improved or did not affect the quality of care within the state.[133]

The health reform plan also made major inroads with regards to cohorts that are usually the least likely to be insured, that is the nonelderly adults and low income residents. Non elderly adults are one of the segments of the least uninsured in USA. About 13.2 million or 29% of the young adult population were without health insurance coverage as of 2007. Usually young adults are dropped from public health insurance or their parents' health insurance policies by the time they turn 19 years old or upon graduation from high school. Some young adults that go on to attend university might get some health insurance coverage but they lose that upon graduation from college as well. This subsequent lack of consistency and stability in coverage puts the health of young adults at risk, while increasing the financial risks of the young adults and their families, just when they are starting out in the workforce.[134] The state of Massachusetts had a high rate of employer provided health insurance prior to the health reform law, but the reform plan helped increase the health insurance coverage of nonelderly adults, though they are still the most uninsured of the state, comprising about 94.5% of the total 120,000 uninsured within the state.[135] The other segment of usually uninsured included low income residents or families earning less than 300% of the Federal Poverty Level (FPL). In MA, this segment comprised 72% of the remaining uninsured and only 40% of the insured population. This group also made appreciable gain in obtaining health insurance coverage after implementation of the health care reform. Out of the total 120,000 uninsured after implementation of the health reform, 72.1% earned less than 300% of the FPL.[136]

The Massachusetts health reform experience shows that, on the whole the individual mandate portion of the health care plan went exceedingly well. About 95% of tax filers complied with the mandate by having insurance year round, while the majority of the 4.2 million tax filers (about 97%) compiled with the state law requirement to file yearly information on their health insurance status. Of the uninsured tax filers, the majority of them, about 76%, were exempt from individual mandate because of their poverty level, that is they were below 150% of the FPL, and had the inability to afford coverage or because they had religious exemption. During calendar year 2008, only about 2% of tax filers were uninsured for part of the year, while only about 4 % were uninsured throughout the year. The tax filers that were subject to the mandate, had less than 1.2% of them assessed a penalty on their 2008 tax return.[137]

Likewise the study of the reform effort indicated that under the law, Employer offer rates of health insurance coverage had increased while that of the rest of the nation remained stagnant. At the same time there was no evidence of government subsidized health insurance crowding out or displacing Employer Sponsored Insurance, there was still a strong employee take up of Employer sponsored health insurance. As a matter of fact, a lot of the employers within the state were utilizing Federal Section 125 tax provisions that allowed employers to purchase health insurance on a pre-tax basis. The state law required employers with 11 or more employees, i.e. about 12% of all employers in MA, to offer a section 125 health plan, and the health plans were subjected to Fair Share Requirements, whereby the employers were required to make "fair and Reasonable" contributions to their employees' health insurance plans. [138]

The state likewise achieved an appreciable degree of success with regards to employers or firms that passed the fair share test. For the initial couple of years after implementation of the reform effort, more than 95% of filing firms met the requirements of the test. During the first year of implementation in 2007, 1020 firms did not meet the requirements of the fair share test, and thus were penalized $10.4 million, whereas for FY 2008, 758 firms were not in compliance and were assessed $7.1 million.[139]

Since the implementation of Massachusetts health reform plan, there had been an appreciable decline in unmet health care needs due to cost within the state, likewise there was significantly increased adults with a regular/consistent source of care, general increased access to care for all adults with concomitant increase in the use of doctors, preventive care and dental services.

Adults at the low to medium income level reported less out of pocket health care expenses, and there was decreased unmet need for care across both middle and low income as well as across minority racial, ethnic and chronically ill population groups. There was also significant reduction across racial and ethnic disparities in access and use of care.[140] This is very impressive because generally within the United States there is a significant health care disparity across racial lines. Different studies have alluded to this health care disparity across racial and ethnic groups. Blacks, Hispanics and Asian adults are generally more likely to be without a usual or regular doctor than white adults. Lack of access is especially acute for Hispanics and blacks. These two ethnic groups are much less likely than adult whites to utilize private physicians as their source of Care. Hispanics usually utilize Community health centers, while blacks are more likely than whites to utilize emergency departments as their regular place of care.[141]

There are differing factors that have been extrapolated as to the reasons why some of these disparities to access to care exist. There is a role that could be attributed to community as well as geographical factors, in which location of domicile plays a role in access to care and subsequently where minority and white individuals seek out care. It is feasible that private physicians might not be opportune or willing to locate to poor communities thus leaving hospital emergency departments and Community health centers as the only viable care location alternatives for minority populations. Barrier to care, can lead to lack of care. According to a 2006 study, almost half of all Hispanics reported that they did not always get needed care, compared with 43 percent of blacks and 41 percent of whites.[142] Likewise Asians are also likely to forgo care, but blacks are more likely than both whites and Hispanics to report delaying or forgoing dental care and prescription drugs.[143] This could have a substantial impact on the quality of their health and the eventual outcome of their health prognosis.

This health care disparity could possibly be attributed to income and health insurance more so than race. It is rather difficult for low income, uninsured individuals to obtain health care services because of the high cost of health care services and as such, the individuals would tend to forgo such health services.[144] The health reform plan in Massachusetts was able to reduce this documented racial and ethnic health care access disparity within their state after implementation of the 2006 health reform plan. Since the health care reform, racial and ethnic disparities in access and utilization of health care have all but disappeared within the state. The general unmet care needs due to costs, for the state dropped dramatically after the reform plan and it fell between 30 and 40% amongst low-income residents and residents with chronic health care conditions. Likewise for the uninsured, there has been an improvement to access to care and barriers to care have decreased since 2006. Generally, now more Massachusetts adults have a usual source of care and utilization of preventive health care services, as well as other health care services has increased.[145] This is very important in managing chronic conditions because preventive care as well as a usual source of care can go a long way to better managing chronic conditions such as hypertension, diabetes, high cholesterol, asthma etc. In the long run, preventive medical services would cut down on use of Emergency departments which would subsequently help cut down on health care costs.

Since the years following the implementation of the reform plan in Massachusetts, public approval within the state has been high for the reform plan and this public approval is consistent across differing ethnic, economic and age groups. There is high physician support for the reform. About 75% of physicians surveyed believed that the reform should be continued, 79% of them believed that the reform helped the previously uninsured and 88% of the physicians believed that the reform improved, or did not affect the care or quality of care provided. Also, the majority of employers concurred that the reform has been good for the state.[146]

While the reform effort had been well received and studies showed that it had improved access to care, there were still some challenges that the reform efforts did not completely addressed. For instance there were still continued barriers to access for some within the state, and there were still some pockets of young non elderly individuals within the state that may be more difficult to convince to purchase health insurance, especially if they are not qualified for government subsidized or employer sponsored health insurance coverage. There was also the issue of increasing health care costs, which despite the reform efforts continued to rise and could threaten the sustainability of the state's health care system.[147] While United States has the highest per capita health care expenditure rate out of all the industrialized countries, the state of Massachusetts has the highest health care costs of any state within U.S.A. and the costs are expected to increase if nothing is done to check the growing costs of health care within the state. Per Capita health care spending for the state is projected to nearly double between now and 2020 if there is no intervention.[148] Nonetheless, it can be feasibly concluded that the Massachusetts health care reform plan was an innovative bold step forward towards the goal of universal coverage for individuals within the state and provision of care, while trying to address cost issues attendant to provision of care.

President Obama's Administration had indicated that the Massachusetts plan, especially the individual mandate of the plan, was the basis for the Patient Protection and Affordable Care Act.[149]

In order to comprehend, the pathway that finally culminated in the Patient Protection and Affordable Care Act it is important to briefly trace the origin and historical development of health services within United States. This will provide some sort of background on the issue of increasing health care costs both at the federal and state levels and why the national health care reform effort was implemented with the end goals of expanding health insurance coverage, while at the same time simultaneously trying to keep cost of provision of quality health care services down.

---

1. Inglehart, J. K. (1994). Health Policy Report: Health Care Reform by the State. Journal of Medicine 330, no. 1, 75-79.
2. Ibid; Mariner, W. (1992). Problems with Employer-Provided Health Insurance: The Employee Retirement Income Security Act and Health Care Reform. New England Journal of Medicine 327, 1682-1685; The Hawaii Prepaid Health Care Act. (n.d.). State of Hawaii, pp. Section 393: 1-53.
3. Ibid
4. McWherter, N. (1993). TennCare: A New Direction in Health Care. Nashville: State of Tennessee Report
5. Ibid
6. Bonneyman, G. (1996). Status of TennCare. Nashville: Center for Health Care Strategies
7. General Accounting Office. (1990). State and Local Finances: Some Jurisdictions Confronted by Short and Long Term Problems. Washington, D.C.: General Accounting Office.
8. McWherter

9. Cromwell, J., Adamache, K. W., Ammering, C., Bartosch, W. J., & Boulis, A. (1995). Equity of the Medicaid Program to the Poor Versus Taxpayers. Health Care Financing Review, 75-104.

10. According to Cromwell et al. in "Equity of the Medicaid Program to the Poor Versus Taxpayers." The standard for Tennessee Aid to Families with Dependent Children (AFDC) program is lower than that for 46 other states in the union.

11. State and Local Finances: Some Jurisdictions Confronted by Short and Long Term Problems.

12. McWherter

13. Ibid

14. Ibid

15. Bonneyman

16. Chase, C. (1998). Changing State and Federal Payment Policies for Medicaid Disproportionate-Share Hospitals. Health Affairs.

17. Coughlin, T., & Liska, D. (1997). The Medicaid Disproportionate Share Hospital Payment Program: Background and Issues. The Urban Institute, no. A-14.

18. Ibid

19. Chase

20. Ibid

21. Prior to enactment of the law, Tennessee as well as several other states in United States had managed to curb escalating health care costs by the use of "Creative Financing techniques, such as disproportionate-share hospital (DSH) payment subsidies as well as other enhanced provider payments.

22. The term "held harmless," as far as DSH payments are concerned, indicate that the providers that paid these taxes or that provided the donations were not going to be harmed financially." In other words they were at least going to get back the initial amount that they had donated or paid as taxes. But with this 1991 law, providers could no longer be guaranteed DSH payments that were at least equal to their taxes or donations. So taxes had to be "real assessments' and donations had to be "bonafide."

23. Ku, L., & Coughlin, T. (1995). Medicaid Disproportionate Share and Other Special Financing Programs. Health Care Financing Review 16, no. 3, 1-54

24. Hudson, T. (1992). States Scramble for Solutions Under New Medicaid Law. Hospitals 66, no. 11, 52-55.

25. Chase

26. Watson, S. D. (1995). Medicaid Physician Participation: Patients, Poverty, and Physician Self Interest. American Journal of Law and Medicine no. 42, 142-151.

27. Coughlin and Liska

28. Ibid

29. Ibid

30. Chase

31. In William Cleverly, Essentials of Health Care Finance (Rockville, MD Aspen Systems Corporation, 1978), 134-158. This can refer to indirect medical education adjustment or allowance that is given to a teaching hospital. This allowance is related to the hospital bed size as well as the number of interns and residents at the hospital. The allowance is usually over and above salaries paid to interns and residents. The adjustment is meant to cover the additional costs incurred by the teaching hospital in the treatment of patients. Hospitals that treat a large percentage of Medicare and Medicaid patients also get a separate payment. This payment is referred to as the disproportionate payment.

32. Hudson

33. Inter-government transfers are fund exchanges between or among different levels of government, such as state or county governments.

34. Chase

35. Ibid

36. Coughlin and Liska

37. Ibid

38. Chase

39. Ibid

40. Ku and Coughlin

41. Coughlin and Liska

42. Before any state can reform the way its Medicaid program is administered, it has to obtain a research and demonstration waiver from HCFA. HCFA is the federal agency that is in charge of administering Medicare and overseeing states' administration of Medicaid. The organization is also responsible for publishing reports on plan performance and reviewing Medicare HMO applications. (Rognnehaugh, R. (1998). The Managed Health Care Dictionary 2nd ed. Gaithersburg, Maryland: Aspen Publishers, Inc.).

43. Lutz, S. (1995). For Real Reform, Watch the States. Modern Healthcare 25, 4: 30-33

44. Ibid

45. Ibid

46. Bonneyman

47. Mirivis, D. M., Chang, C. F., Hall, C. J., Zaar, G. T., & Applegate, W. B. (1995). TennCare: Health System Reform for Tennessee. Journal of the American Medical Association 274, 15: 1235

48. McWherter

49. Ibid

50. Ibid

51. TennCare Standard was usually for individuals that could afford to pay a monthly premium but were not eligible for TennCare Medicaid. It should be noted not everyone on the standard could afford to pay a premium. These are usually individuals that are uninsured, uninsurable, or medically ineligible. According to the mandate, by April 2005, adults over 19 were no longer eligible for TennCare Standard. (TennCare Information)

52 . TennCare Information. (2006). Retrieved December 15, 2010, from THA: http://www.tha.com/pdffiles/THA-Legisl-Conf-2006/2006-TennCare-Reform.pdf

53. Ibid

54. Aid to Families with Dependent Children was replaced in TN by Families first. The program offers temporary cash assistance while emphasizing work, training and personal responsibility. Since the program had a maximum lifetime assistance of 60 months, participants were expected to gradually wean themselves off the program (there were specific exceptions and exemptions).

55. TennCare Information

56. NCQA is an independent non-profit organization that rates managed care organization's performance with regards to utilization management, provider credentials, quality improvement and member rights and responsibilities.

57. HEDIS stands for Health Plan Employer Data and Information Set, and it is a measure that allows consumers to compare managed care performance across several indicators.

58. Gordon, D., Long, W., & Killingsworth, P. (2010). TennCare Oversight Committee Presentation. Retrieved April 4, 2011, from http://www.capitol.tn.gov/joint/committees/ tenncare/tenncareoversight082410.pdf

59. Ibid
60. Brown, L. (1991). The National Politics of Oregon's Rationing Plan. Health Affairs 10, no. 2, 28-51; and Fox, D., & Leichter, H. (1991). Rationing Care in Oregon: The New Accountability. Retrieved August 12, 2012, from Health Affairs: http://content.healthaffairs.org/content/10/2/7.full.pdf+html?ijkey=1f3dfa96d8992408f18 69b3e4f449f942b34613d&keytype2=tf_ipsecsha
61. Oberlander, J. (2007). Health Reform Interrupted: The Unraveling of the Oregon Health Plan. Retrieved August 7, 2010, from Health Affairs: http://content.healthaffairs.org/content/26/1/w96.full
62. Ibid
63 . Oregon Health Plan. (n.d). Retrieved August 8, 2012 from Oregon.gov: http://cms.oregon.gov/oha/healthplanpages/priorlist/main.aspx
64. Ibid
65. Brown
66. Ibid
67. Ibid
68. Ibid
69. Ibid
70. Oberlander
71. Bonneyman, in "Status of TennCare," indicated that the normal lack of medical care often culminated in increased emergency room visits for ailments that sometimes were not critical in nature.
72. Reinhardt, U. (2009, July 3). Rationing, Health Care: What Does it Mean? Retrieved August 10, 2012, from New York Times: http://economix.blogs.nytimes.com/2009/07/03 /rationing-health-care-what-does-it-mean/ ; and Katz, M., & Rosen, H. (1997) in Micro-economics 3rd Edition, McGraw Hill/ Irwin Publishers
73. Ibid
74. Ibid
75. Schoen, C., Osborn, R., How, S. K., Doty, M. M., & Peugh, J. (2008). *In Chronic Conditions: Experiences of Patients With Complex Health Care Needs in Eight Countries.* Retrieved 2012, from Health Affairs: http://content.healthaffairs.org/content/ 28/1/w1.full.pdf+html?sid=274e8699-1920-4065-a257-1ff2ea0d80f3
76. Hadley, J., Holahan, J., Coughlin, T., & Miller, D. (2008, August 25). Covering the Unisured in 2008: Current Cost, Sources of Payment, and Incremental Cost. *Health Affairs 27, no. 5*
77. Abelson, R. (2009, June 30). Insured but Bankrupted by Health Crisis. Retrieved August 10, 2012, from The New York Times: http://www.nytimes.com/2009/07/01/ business/01meddebt.html?_r=1#
78. *Hidden Cost Value Lost, Uninsurance in America.* (2003). Retrieved August 10, 2012, from Institute of Medicine (IOM): http://books.nap.edu/openbook.php?record_id= 10719&page=R2
79. Reinhardt, U. (2009, July 3). Rationing, Health Care: What Does it Mean? Retrieved August 10, 2012, from New York Times: http://economix.blogs.nytimes.com/2009/07/03 /rationing-health-care-what-does-it-mean
80. Horsley, S. (2012, August 9). Doctors Say Health Care Rationing Already Exists. Retrieved August 9, 2012, from National Public Radio:http://www.npr.org/templates/ story/story.php?storyId=106168331.
81. Ibid
82. Ibid

83. Ibid
84. Brown
85. Fox and Leichter
86. Ibid
87. Oberlander
88. Fox and Leichter
89. Ibid
90. Local Area Unemplyment Statistics: General Overview. (n.d.). Retrieved November 29, 2006, from U.S. Department of Labor, Bureau of Labor Statistics:http://www.bls.gov/lau/home.htm#overview
91. 1115 Waiver Amendment Application. (2002, May 21). State of Oregon.
92. Brown
93. Oberlander
94. Ibid
95. Conis, E., & Medlin, C. (2008, November). Update on Oregon Health Plan (OHP) Restructuring. Retrieved August 12, 2012, from http://hpm.org/en/Surveys/IGH_-_USA/11/Update_on_Oregon_Health_Plan_%28OHP%29_Restructuring.html
96. Oberlander
97. Conis and Medlin
98. Ibid
99. Oberlander
100. Ibid
101. Ibid
115. Conis and Medlin
103. Ibid
104. Ibid
105. Ibid
106. Ibid
107. Bill Graves, Gov. John Kitzhaber wants to give Oregon Health Plan a boost with better, less costly care. (Oregon Live. (2011, April 7). Retrieved August 13, 2012 from: http://www.oregonlive.com/health/index.ssf/2011/04/gov_john_kitzhaber_wants_to_gi.html)
108. Ibid
109 . Coordinated Care Organizations. (n.d.). Retrieved August 13, 2012, from Oregon.gov: http://cms.oregon.gov/oha/ohpb/pages/health-reform/ccos.aspx
110. Ibid
111. Ibid
112. Ibid
113. Ibid
114. Hirschkorn, P., & Glor, J. (2012, June 24). Massachusetts' Health Care Plan: 6 years Later. Retrieved August 13, 2012, from CBS News: http://www.cbsnews.com/8301-18563_162-57459563/massachusetts-health-care-plan-6-years-later/
115. It must be noted that short gaps in coverage, about three months or less are allowed without attendant penalties.
116. Massachusetts Health Insurance Requirements. (2012). Retrieved August 14, 2012, from MassResources.org: http://www.massresources.org/health-reform.html#reformact
117. Ibid
118. A qualified employer or self-employed person is defined by MassHealth, as an employer that has no more than 50 employees and provides health insurance for the employ-

ees that meet the basic requirements of MassHealth. The employer must also pay at least 50% of the premium cost for the insurance provided for the employees and take part within the Insurance Partnership program.

119. MassHealth defines an adult caretaker relative as an adult relative living with a child under 19 within the same home and is the primary caretaker or caregiver of the child. The child's parents are not present within the home, and the child could be related to the caretaker by blood, adoption or marriage or is the spouse or former spouse of one of those relatives.

120. Long term care is defined by MassHealth as the care needed by an individual who is not able to care for him/herself over a long period due to chronic disease or disability. This would include care within the individual's home, a nursing home or assisted living facility.

121. MassHealth: General Eligibility Requirements. (2012). Retrieved August 14, 2012, from MassResources.org: http://www.massresources.org/masshealth-general-eligibility.html

122. Massachusetts Health Insurance Requirements

123. Ibid

124. Ibid

125. Health Connector Commonwealth Care Program Guide. (2012). Retrieved August 19, 2012, from https://www.mahealthconnector.org/portal/binary/com.epicentric.content management.servlet.ContentDeliveryServlet/About%2520Us/CommonwealthCare/Com monwealth%2520Care%2520Program%2520Guide.pdf

126. Commonwealth Care. (2012). Retrieved August 15, 2012, from MassResources.org: http://www.massresources.org/commonwealth-care.html#incomelimits

127. Ibid

128. Health Connector Commonwealth Care Program Guide. (2012). Retrieved August 19, 2012, https://www.mahealthconnector.org/portal/binary/com.epicentric.content management.servlet.ContentDeliveryServlet/About%2520Us/CommonwealthCare/Com monwealth%2520Care%2520Program%2520Guide.pdf

129. Ibid

130. Commonwealth Care

131. Massachusetts Health Insurance Requirements

132 . Health Reform in Massachusetts: Expaninding Access to Health Insurance Coverage: Assessing the Results. (2011, April). Retrieved August 17, 2012, from Blue Cross Blue Shield Massachusetts Foundation: http://bluecrossmafoundation.org/Health-Reform/~/media/D0DDA3D667BE49D58539821F74C723C7.pdf

133. Ibid

134. Nicholson, J. L., Collins, S. R., Mahato, B., Gould, E., Schoen, C., & Rustgi, S. D. (2009). Rite of Passage? Why Young Adults Become Uninsured and How New Policies Can Help. Retrieved August 17, 2012, from The CommonWealth Fund Issue Brief: http://www.commonwealthfund.org/~/media/Files/Publications/Issue%20Brief/2009/Aug /1310_Nicholson_rite_of_passage_2009.pdf

135. Health Reform in Massachusetts: Expanding Access to Health Insurance Coverage: Assessing the Results

136. Ibid

137. Ibid

138. Ibid

139. Ibid

140. Ibid

141. Mead, H., Cartwright-Smith, L., Jones, K., Ramos, C., Woods, K., & Siegel, B. (2008). Racial and Ethnic Disparities in U.S Health Care: A Chart Book, Vol. 27.
142. Ibid
143. Ibid
144. Ibid
145. Health Reform in Massachusetts: Expanding Access to Health Insurance Coverage: Assessing the Results
146. Ibid
147. Ibid
148. Ibid
149. Hirschkorn and Glor

Chapter 3

A Brief History of the Financing, Costing and Economics of Health Care in the United States

There have been various efforts since the twentieth century within United States to provide some sort of universal health insurance coverage to its citizens. Prior to the turn of the 20th century, the United States government had no program to subsidize or help individuals pay for their health care costs. Basically the federal government let the states decide what to do with regards to caring for their sick, and the states in turn let private and voluntary organizations decide how to help care for indigent patients. There were no legislative or public programs during the period spanning the late 19th through the early 20th century, but United States did have some voluntary funds that provided for congressional members in cases of sickness or death.[1] Apart from that, individuals were expected to pay for the costs of their medical services. These services were usually provided by both physicians and nurses. Those that could not afford to pay for private physicians and medications had to utilize charitable institutions. These institutions were established as voluntary, nonprofit corporations that provided charity health care for indigent patients.

During President Theodore Roosevelt's Progressive Era, most of the initiatives for health care reform were outside the realm of government despite the fact that President Roosevelt supported the idea of health insurance, since he believed that no country would truly be strong if its people were sick and poor.[2] During this period the American Association of Labor Legislation (AALL), a typical progressive group led the push for health insurance. The focus of the AALL was on reforming rather than abolishing capitalism. They formed a committee in 1912 and subsequently decided to focus on health insurance issues and ended up drafting a model bill in 1915. The bill was to provide health insurance coverage to working class citizens that earned less than $1,200/year. The coverage would also cover their dependents and provide for payment of services of physicians, nurses, hospitals as well as cover sick pay, maternity benefits, and a funereal expense death benefit of fifty dollars. The proposed health insurance costs were to be borne between workers, employers, and the state.[3] The American Medical Association (AMA) initially supported the AALL proposal but since there were repeated denouncements of compulsory health insurance by the president of the American Federation of Labor (AFL), the initial AMA support eroded. The president of AFL derided compulsory health insurance as an unnecessary paternalistic reform that would create an unwanted system of state supervision over people's health. The main fear was that unions would be weakened, since their roles in providing social benefits would be overshadowed by a government based health insurance system. Likewise the commercial insurance industry opposed the idea of a government health insurance program. Inherent and central to the commercial insurance business was the death benefits that covered funeral expenses paid by the working poor to ensure that they did not have a "Pauper's burial." The proposed government health insurance would likewise cover death benefits thus negating the need for the working class to buy commercial death benefits. This would have significantly affected the profits of the commercial insurance industry, thus they were vehemently opposed to the idea of government sponsored health insurance.[4]

With the onset of World War 1 in 1917, and the subsequent anti German sentiment during that period, opponents of government health insurance linked the idea of government health insurance to "German Socialist Insurance" inconsistent with American Values. This helped put an end to the initial discourse about government health insurance during this era.[5] The beginning of the 20th century also saw the development of city/county hospitals, which were established by local governments to provide care for indigent patients in their areas or locales. These indigent patients could not pay for their own care nor obtain the services of the charity hospitals.[6] These hospitals were usually large acute care facilities with busy clinics and emergency rooms with close connections to local government ambulance services, police department and other community services. During the same period, state governments also began to assume responsibility for the care of the insane.[7]

After World War II there was a surge in health care costs, with resultant increase in development and the variety of health insurance plans. The post-war period saw the development of community based non-profit Blue Cross/Blue Shield plans,[8] and labor union health and welfare trust funds. These funds were established as a result of benefit negotiations for union members. During this period, private for profit commercial insurance companies increased their scope of efforts for the benefit of their beneficiaries. Their beneficiaries included both individuals and large groups of employees. It was within this period that different and large government sponsored and publicly managed insurance health care plans evolved, such as Medicare and Medicaid.[9]

The growth or increase of these health insurance plans seemed to occur in tandem with development of private medical practitioners, city and state government hospitals, voluntary nonprofit hospitals as well as military and veteran hospitals. This variety in the provision of health care seemed suited for United States with its wide diversity of people and situations.[10] The period encompassing 1945 through 1970 was rife with developments in United States health care.[11] There was the push during Truman's Presidency (1945-1953) for universal comprehensive health insurance coverage that was egalitarian in nature and would include all classes of society and not just for the needy. He tried to make the pitch that comprehensive health insurance coverage was not "socialized medicine." In order to try and gain more support and approval for his universal insurance idea, President Truman dropped the funeral benefit that was crucial to the defeat of the AALL proposal. There was not much congressional support for this proposal as well. The House Committee Chairman was an anti-union conservative and subsequently refused to hold hearings, meanwhile Republican Senator Taft suggested that compulsory health insurance strictly originated from the soviet constitution and he stated, "I consider it socialism. It is to my mind the most socialistic measure this Congress has ever had before it,"[12] and he subsequently walked out of the hearings. Likewise the American Medical Association (AMA), the American Hospital Association, the American Bar Association, and the majority of the press hated the plan. Despite the fact that President Truman had emphasized that doctors would be able to choose their method of payment, the AMA claimed that it would make doctors slaves.[13]

Subsequently Republicans took control of Congress in 1946, and were not interested in the idea of a universal government health insurance claiming that the idea was part of a larger socialist scheme. Despite the opposition to his plan President Truman ran for reelection by focusing on a national health bill, and won reelection in 1948. The AMA thought his reelection was Armageddon and this spurred the AMA into an aggressive and expensive lobbying effort to defeat the idea of a national health insurance plan. AMA members were charged $25 extra and in 1945 AMA spent about $1.5 million on lobbying efforts against the national health plan. One of their pamphlets read as follows;

"Would socialized medicine lead to socialization of other phases of life? Lenin thought so. He declared socialized medicine is the keystone to the arch of the socialist state." [14]

This ability to link the idea of universal comprehensive government sponsored health plan to socialism was very effective and with the anti-Communist sentiment of the late 1940's Korean War era, President Truman's health plan subsequently died in congressional committee. The private health insurance plans that were in existence for those who could afford it expanded and became the norm, while the poor had public welfare services. Likewise Union-negotiated health care benefits were available for workers and that helped starve off concentrated efforts for a government program.[15]

These developments were governed by mutual interests between insurers and providers who formed a sort of coalition that allowed for flow of funds from payers of care to insurers, providers and suppliers of health care.[16] These funds helped promote scientific progress in the field of medicine.[17] After 1970 there were obvious signs of deteriorating United States economy, while simultaneously health care costs were rapidly increasing. The increasing health care costs were spurred by great strides in intricate and costly biotechnological development and the public's desire to utilize expensive most advanced treatment and diagnostic techniques. Thus deterioration of United States economy and rapid increase in health care expenditures clashed with the need for biotechnological development and the public's desire for advanced diagnostic techniques and treatment. This was a major factor in spiraling health care costs. The major payers i.e. government and business, tried to stem the growth of health care funding. This led to an uneasy relationship between insurers and providers of care thus straining their alliance, while opening the health care sector to immense political and economic change.[18] Bodenhimer and Grumbach indicated that:

> As the payers limited which insurers and providers would receive payments, competition intensified within the health care industry with the big-large insurers, large hospitals, and large physician groups gaining ascendancy over the small. Selective contracting gives payers a great deal of power because they can deny contracts with insurers and providers who fail to keep costs down. The heightened power of the payers has led to a new relationship between insurers and providers. First, HMOs merge insurers and providers into one organization; thus, insurers owning HMOs also function as providers of care. Second, within insurer-controlled HMOs, the insurers play the role of managers while the true providers-hospitals and physicians -are the direct producers of medical services. In some cases, HMOs own hospitals and employ physicians. In other cases, HMOS determine which hospitals and physicians will receive their patients and how much those providers will be paid.[19]

Therefore providers no longer had full autonomy in determining their fees. This lack of full autonomy had spawned a system where insurers now virtually call the shots in determining how much providers could be paid for their services.

There are different participants, within the trillion-dollar health care industry, but Thomas Bodenhimer and Kevin Grumbach emphasize that modern day health care stage is comprised of four major actors. These actors are:

1) The payers who supply the money to pay for utilized health care. The payers would include individuals[20] that utilize health care services, businesses that pay for their employees' health insurance and government since it provides payment for care through public programs such as Medicare and Medicaid;

2) The insurers who take money from payers, assume risk, and then pay providers when policy holders need medical care. So insurers basically receive money from payers and utilize some of the money to reimburse providers;[21]

3) Providers who are the individuals or organizations that actually provides the health care;

4) Suppliers would refer to the pharmaceutical and medical supply industries that provide health care equipment, supplies and medications utilized by providers in treating patients.[22] These different

participants are interconnected in the insurance, management and provision of health services.

It is necessary to understand the interrelationship between these participants so as to have a basic comprehension of the health care process within United States. There is an underlying tension between payers/insurers of health care and members of the health care industry i.e. providers and suppliers of health care. Whenever the payer or insurer spends money for health care it represents income to the health care industry. Payers wish to contain their costs, while providers and suppliers of health care wish to see an increase in the amount of money spent on health care.

It is difficult to specify with any degree of certainty a particular proven or consistent modus operandi of health care in United States. It would seem that new and different ideas predominate for a while within the health care field but with passage of time, these ideas appear not to work nor produce any sort of solution to the problem of providing quality and cost efficient health care. Hence the general perspective is that the health care field goes through periods of evolution in the process of trying to attain an optimum goal, whereby every citizen would have quality health coverage at a reasonable cost. The changes undergone by the health care field in United States would include shifting from payment of services rendered to buying into indemnity type insurance plans (which pay providers on a fee for service basis), to federal government involvement in paying for health insurance plans. Currently there is an emphasis on Managed Care plans that advocate some sort of implicit rationing of health care in the pursuit of reduced health care costs. All these changes came about when it seemed that the former way of payment and provision of services did not appear to provide adequate health coverage at a reasonable price.

These changes or revolutions could be likened to Thomas Kuhn's assertions about scientific revolutions.[23] The author's assertions imply that if a paradigm can no longer solve "problems," then there is the tendency for the paradigm to be replaced with another. In other words the old paradigm is seen as being "insufficient" and this consequently leads to "scientific revolutions." These revolutions are considered the result of a "crisis." According to the author:

> The transition from a paradigm in crisis to a new one from which a new tradition of normal science can emerge is far from a cumulative process, one achieved by an articulation or extension of the old paradigm. Rather it is a reconstruction of the field from new fundamentals, a reconstruction that changes some of the field's most elementary theoretical generalizations as well as many of its paradigm methods and applications. During the transition period there will be a large but never complete overlap between the problems that can be solved by the old and by the new paradigm. But there will also be a decisive difference in the modes of solution. When the transition is complete, the profession will have changed its view of the field, its methods, and its goals.[24]

The above process could be visualized within context of the health care industry, whereby the industry appears to have gone through so many transitions in trying to find a cost effective and efficient means of providing health care. These transitions would include as mentioned before, focusing on indemnity type plans and then shifting focus from such plans to managed care plans. The transitions and changes could also be perceived in terms of reimbursement, which has run the gamut from reimbursement based on charges, to reimbursement based on hospital costs, to Diagnosis Related Group (DRG) reimbursement[25] methods and to what is currently most common, that is reimbursement based on predetermined rates by managed care organizations.

There is no single or easily described American system of health care; instead there are four models or subsystems of health care in America, each of which serve a different group of individuals. Accordingly these systems serve the following different groups:

1) Regularly employed, middle-income families with continuous programs of health insurance coverage;
2) Poor, unemployed (or underemployed) families without continuous health insurance coverage;
3) Active-duty military personnel and their dependents; and
4) Veterans of United States military service.[26]

A similar view of the United States frame work for health insurance can be broken down into three categories which reflect to some extent the employment status of individuals within the insurance program. These categories would include: Voluntary Health Insurance (VHI), which is usually private insurance that covers current industrial employees; Social Health Insurance (SHI), which indicates participation in a government entitlement program that is linked to prior employment and finally; Public Welfare programs which are for individuals that do not have employment, have low income employment or are unable to gain employment due to disability.[27]

These above two schemas for classifying the United States health system recognize the significance of no insurance for the unemployed or underemployed, though it does not take into consideration the uninsurable that is those individuals with chronic diseases. Their chronic diseases make it almost impossible for them to purchase new affordable health insurance plans on their own, because their chronic diseases would usually be classified as preexisting conditions, and health insurance companies prior to the Patient Protection and Affordable care Act were loath to provide coverage for preexisting conditions.

This book also focuses on the uninsured or uninsurable due to preexisting medical conditions. This is because PPACA was signed mainly to address insurance coverage for the aforementioned population as well as expand scope of services to the general population regardless of preexisting conditions.

Background on Medicare and Medicaid

Medicare was instituted as part of Social Security Amendments of 1965, which established two separate but coordinated health insurance plans for persons aged 65 or older. The first part is known as part A of Medicare and it is the compulsory program of hospital insurance (HI), which provides hospital insurance for qualified individuals. The second part is B, and it is a voluntary program of Supplementary Medical Insurance (SMI). The SMI was intended to complement the HI program. As such it provided necessary payment for physician's services, outpatient services as well as rural and home health visits for individuals without Part A. Medicare was subsequently amended in 1972 to provide coverage for certain severely disabled persons under the age of 65 and to individuals suffering from end stage renal disease. This was in addition to providing general coverage for individuals over the age of 60.[28]

Initially, Medicare was operated as a fee for service plan for physicians and related services. Then, Medicare hospital reimbursement was based on any reasonable costs incurred in provision of covered medical care to Medicare patients. But with increasing costs, reimbursement format was changed in 1983, to a prospective payment system, whereby rates were determined on a case by case basis, using diagnosis-related groups (DRGs) to classify cases for reimbursement.[29] The DRG is a Yale University-derived system of classification for 383 inpatient hospital services that were based on principal diagnosis, secondary diagnosis, surgical procedures, sex, age and the presence of complications. So, DRG classification is therefore utilized as a basis for compensating hospitals and other providers.[30] The cost of Medicare had been increasing, therefore the Tax Equity and Fiscal Responsibility Act of 1982 (TEFRA) was implemented. This law was enacted with the goal of setting limits on reimbursements of hospital costs at the per case level and also limited the annual rate of increase for Medicare's reasonable costs per discharge.[31] Major components of the law, included revisions to the Medicare law to encourage growth in number of Health Maintenance Organizations (HMO) and other comprehensive medical plans that enroll Medicare beneficiaries.[32]

Medicaid was enacted into law on July 30, 1965 as a Title XIX program of the Social Security Act..[33] Prior to enactment of Medicaid, states and local governments took care of the poor in their respective locales. In some instances doctors donated their services or assessed indigent patient's charges for services on a sliding scale. But with enactment of Medicaid, the program became part of existing federal-state welfare structure.[34] Therefore, Medicaid was initially planned as a medical care extension of federally funded income maintenance programs for the poor with a focus on provision of care for dependent children and their mothers.[35] Since Medicaid is welfare medicine, it has no entitlement features, so recipients must prove their eligibility according to their monthly or yearly income. Medicaid eligibility criteria and services provided are complex and vary considerably among states. Services can change within a state during the year and also one [36]can be eligible for certain services in one state but would not be eligible in another state. This is because the states have autonomy in choosing their criteria for eligibility. There is a great deal of variability within state standards for income and asset levels for cash assistance and medical eligibility. It is also within the authority of states to determine scope of services provided.[37]

Since its inception the Medicaid program has been operated as a vendor payment system, which was designed to provide more effective medical care for individuals that needed it. This was to be achieved through improved standards of care, liberal eligibility rules and increased federal matching under a formula with no limit.[38]

Medicaid is welfare medicine whereas Medicare is a form of social health insurance (SHI). Within that context Medicaid is a transfer payment 'in kind" which implies that medical services are provided as a welfare benefit instead of cash. Cash subsides are also provided for welfare recipients to pay for their living expenses, although their medical benefits are paid directly to the providers so as to make it impossible for recipients to spend the money on other necessities rather than on health care.[39]

Social health insurance (SHI) on the other hand, is not charity but entitlement program. In that regards it is a right earned by individuals during the period of their employment, when they paid in, into the system. Payroll tax is utilized in funding SHI programs, for example social security is funded by payroll tax which is divided between the worker and employer. Social health insurance programs are supposed to provide members of society with protection against hazards that are so widespread as to be considered risks that individuals cannot afford to deal with on their own. Therefore eligibility in SHI is derived from contributions that have been made into the program by the individuals and benefits are statutory rights, and thus not based on need. Therefore Medicare recipients are entitled to benefits of SHI.[40]

Medicaid spending is one of the fastest growing areas of state spending. In order to try and control costs, different strategies were utilized by different state governments. Such strategies as mentioned previously included prepaid managed health care, utilization review, case management, reimbursement via diagnosis related group (DRG). Other strategies included new services for elderly, disabled and AIDS stricken individuals. Prior to enactment of PPACA, cost containment efforts were focused on shifting Medicaid funding from federal to state budgets while encouraging states to pattern their systems after Health Maintenance Organizations (HMOs).[41] It is interesting to note that the health reform plan that was instituted in Tennessee i.e. TennCare was patterned after HMOs,[42] in that the plan was fundamentally Medicaid being operated as a managed care program. Likewise the Oregon health plan and the Massachusetts health plan utilized some components of managed care plans.

1. Palmer, K. S. (1999). A Brief History: Universal Care Efforts in the US. Retrieved August 19, 2012, from Physicians for a National Health Program: http://www.pnhp.org/facts/a-brief-history-universal-health-care-efforts-in-the-us
2. Ibid
3. Ibid
4. Ibid
5. Ibid
6. Torrens, P. R. (1993). Historical Evolution of Health Services in the United States. In S. J. Williams, & P. R. Torrens, Introduction to Health Services, 4th Edition (pp. 14-28). New York, New York: Delmar Publishers Inc.
7. Ibid
8. According to Paul Torrens, these Blue Cross and Blue shield plans were developed by hospital and physician associations, so as to spread health care costs more widely amongst the population.
9. Torrens
10. Ibid
11. Bodenhimer, T., & Grumbach, K. (1995). The Reconfiguration of U.S. Medicine. The Journal of the American Medical Association 274 no. 1, 85-92.
12. Palmer
13. Bodenhimer and Grumbach
14. Ibid
15. Ibid
16. Ibid
17. Ibid
18. Ibid
19. Ibid
20. It is necessary to mention that individuals are ultimately the payers of all health care because individuals finance both government and businesses by paying taxes and purchasing the products of businesses.
21. Some insurers can also be considered as payers due to the fact that they can also pay for services while also being able to receive money from payers. The government can be viewed in this category when the Medicaid and Medicare programs are considered.
22. Bodenhimer and Grumbach
23. Kuhn, T. (1970). The Structure of Scientific Revolutions 3rd ed. Chicago: The University of Chicago Press.
24. Ibid
25. This is a prospective reimbursement schema whereby health care providers are paid on a predetermined rate or a fixed dollar amount based on diagnosis of the condition being treated. As such diseases are classified into different categories with different payment levels for the different categories of diseases. If the diagnosis is for a cold for instance and the payment rate for that is say $50, then a provider could not be paid more than $50 regardless of cost of providing care to a particular patient that had the cold.
26. Torrens
27. Koch, A. (1993). Financing Health Services. In S. J. Williams, & P. R. Torrens, Introduction to Health Services, 4th Edition (p. 302). New York, New York: Delmar Publishers Inc.
28. Social Security Programs in the United States, Bulletin 56, no. 4. (1993). Washington, D.C.: U.S. Department of Health and Human Services.
29. Koch

30. Rognehaugh, R. (1998). The Managed Health Care Dictionary 2nd ed. Gaithersburg, Maryland: Aspen Publishers, Inc.

31. Koch

32. Ibid

33. Ibid

34. Ibid

35. Social Security Programs in the United States, Bulletin 56, no. 4.

36. This implies that medical services are provided as a welfare benefit instead of cash.

37. Koch

38. Social Security Programs in the United States, Bulletin 56, no. 4.

39. Koch

40. Ibid; Roemer, M. I. (1978). Social Medicine: The Advance of Organized Health Services in America. New York: Springer.

41. Altman, D., & Dennis, B. (1990). Perspectives on the Medicaid Program. Health Care Financing Review 12, 2-5.

42. HMOS utilize medical gatekeepers to ration the use of health care services. These gatekeepers are usually primary care physicians, and they have inbuilt incentives to ration medical care according to HMO's guidelines. This is depending on the particular HMO, the physicians' financial compensations are better when they keep within the HMO guidelines. The covered individual can switch HMOs if the guidelines are not acceptable, but the HMOs' guidelines are mostly determined by the premiums, i.e. HMOs that have more costly premiums usually have more lax rationing rules. This idea is inherent in utilizing managed care for TennCare.

Chapter 4

The Patient Protection and Affordable Health Care Plan

Given, the issues and problems mentioned previously, with provision of coverage for different segments of the population as well as increasing health care costs, the stage was set for a solution to try and address the lack of health coverage and increasing health care costs, especially at the federal level. President Obama's landmark Patient Protection and Affordable Care Act (PPACA) was signed into law on March 23rd 2010. The health care law is a health insurance reform plan that would invariably change the way health care is delivered and paid for within the United States. The majority of the mandates of the health care law are supposed to be carried out by 2014, while the rest would take effect by 2020. It is important to note, that some mandates of the law have already been adopted.

The Health Care Law is one of the most ambitious health care overhaul laws in USA modern history. The law was enacted with the end goal of providing universal health coverage for citizens within USA. As such the law would extend coverage to more than 30 million uninsured individuals, through Medicaid expansion, subsidies and individual mandate. Prior to the enactment of the law, providers and the individual states had to bear the burden of uncompensated care. This put a heavy financial burden on the states. Uninsured individuals usually do not utilize preventive health services or checkups since they could not afford to pay for it. Invariably, when they got very sick or had a medical emergency, they would seek emergency room services. This type of service is generally very expensive, but since legally, within the United States; patients cannot be denied treatment or turned away from a hospital if they are having a medical emergency, the hospitals and subsequently the individual states would bear the uncompensated care cost of the expensive emergency visit.

Much of the controversy surrounding PPACA was on what is commonly known as an individual mandate. This is whereby most adult individuals are required to have private health insurance coverage if they do not have either a government or employer sponsored health insurance, otherwise they would be required to pay a fine. The legislation as signed into law, by Congress, expanded the provision of Medicaid [1] to nearly everyone making up to 133 percent of the federal poverty line. Medicaid is governmental health insurance coverage for indigent people and families, who have limited income and resources. Different States have different rules for determining income so as to determine eligibility for Medicaid. Eligibility may also depend on your age, whether you are a United States citizen,[2] pregnant, blind or have any other disabilities. If Medicaid covers a woman's labor and delivery, it will subsequently cover the child born for up to a year without needing to apply separately for the child.[3]

So the proposed Medicaid expansion under the health reform law was slated to add an estimated 16 million people to state Medicaid coverage within the next seven years. A key part of this provision as written was that States that refused to comply with this expansion, or that preferred to opt out of this, would possibly lose all their Medicaid funding.[4] Opponents of PPACA, see this as mandating individuals to buy something (in this instance health insurance) which they contend is against the constitution. They also see it as taking away the autonomy of the individual states by requiring that they expand their Medicaid rolls otherwise face possibility of losing federal Medicaid funding in cases of noncompliance. The Act likewise precludes insurance companies from utilizing gender or preexisting conditions in determining coverage. As such, all health insurance companies are mandated to offer the same rates to all applicants as well as insure all applicants regardless of health or gender.[5]

The Congressional Budget office, determined, in its reports that the health law would potentially reduce Medicare spending [6] and lower future deficit spending that accrues as a result of lack of health insurance coverage.[7] According to CBO "Through those changes and numerous others, the 2010 legislation significantly decreased Medicare outlays relative to what they would have been under prior law."[8] Thus the report indicated that without the health care reform law, Medicare spending would be much higher.

Regardless, opponents of the health care law, including 28 states, various organizations and private individuals mounted a legal suit, challenging the constitutionality of the law. On June 28, 2012, the Supreme Court of the United States upheld the constitutionality of most mandates of PPACA in *National Federation of Independent Business v. Sebelius.* [9] However, the Supreme Court, ruled against the law's requirement that States that refused to comply with Medicaid expansion, or that preferred to opt out of this expansion, would possibly lose all their Medicaid funding. According to Chief Justice Roberts, writing for the majority, the federal government can attach conditions to the money they wish to provide to the states for such expansion, but to weld the threat of cutting off their regular Medicaid funding if they choose not to opt in, is tantamount to economic "dragooning," which would invariably lead the states with no choice but to opt in. This is especially true when federal Medicaid funding to the states comprise more than 10% of their state budgets. As such the Supreme Court did not uphold that particular section of the law.

Prior to enactment of PPACA about 56 million individuals in USA were covered by Medicaid health insurance.[10] PPACA Medicaid expansion would dramatically increase the number of individuals covered by Medicaid. The Supreme Court had determined in its June 28th 2012 ruling that the federal government could withhold existing money that helped states run their pre-expansion programs, but the Highest court in the land also ruled that the federal government could withhold Medicaid expansion funds for each particular state that wanted to opt out or that did not wish to expand its Medicaid rolls. The states were then left with the choice of determining if they wanted to opt out and not receive the federal expansion funds or opt in and receive the expansion funds. The federal government prior to enactment of the health care law contributed an average of about 57 % of a state's Medicaid funding.[11] All the states within the United States are opted into Medicaid, despite the fact that they can choose not to participate in Medicaid. The expansion indicated by PPACA, would extend Medicaid coverage to almost everyone that makes up to 133 percent of the federal poverty level. Prior to PPACA implementation, many states only covered adults with children if their income was much lower and they did not cover childless adults under Medicaid.

As late as 2010, about 33.3 percent of states did not cover parents with dependent children who were at 100% of the federal poverty level. Likewise only the District of Columbia and six other states offered Medicaid coverage to low income adults without dependent children. The Health Care reform expansion would add an estimated 16 million people to state Medicaid rolls over the subsequent seven year period following enactment of the law.[12] It should be clarified that under the mandates of PPACA, the federal government would cover 100% of State's Medicaid expansion costs for the first three initial years of the law, i.e. from 2014 through 2016, and then subsequently, federal coverage would decline gradually until 2020 and beyond when it would permanently cover costs of the expansion at 90%. This should be contrasted with the average 57 percent Medicaid coverage provided by the federal government prior to enactment of PPACA. It is also important to note that the 28 states (listed in the table below) that joined in filing the lawsuit against the law, account for the country's most unemployed people and likewise account for about 55 percent of the nation's uninsured, which is a total of 27.6 million uninsured people.[13]

Table 4.1- List of States' Attorneys General (or Governors*) Acting to Pursue Lawsuits Opposing Health Provisions. [14]

Alabama	3/23/10
Alaska	4/21/10
Arizona *	4/07/10
Colorado §	3/23/10

Florida	3/23/10
Georgia *	4/13/10
Idaho	3/23/10
Indiana	4/07/10
Iowa **	1/18/11
Kansas	1/18/11
Louisiana	3/23/10
Maine **	1/18/11
Michigan §	3/23/10
Mississippi *	4/07/10
Missouri §§§	3/11
Nebraska	3/23/10
Nevada *	4/07/10
North Dakota	4/07/10
Ohio **	1/18/11
Pennsylvania §§	3/23/10
South Carolina	3/23/10
South Dakota	3/23/10
Texas	3/23/10
Utah	3/23/10
Virginia (1-statsuit)	Appeals 9/08/11
Washington §	3/23/10
Wisconsin **	1/18/11
Wyoming **	1/18/11

* States where legal action was initiated by governors' offices.

** Newly elected executive branch officials for 2011 announced support for lawsuit.

§ States where Attorney General initiated action but Governor publicly supports law opposes challenge.

§§ The Republican AG of Penn. was elected Governor on 11/2/2010.

§§§ Missouri Lieutenant Governor Peter Kinder and six state residents sued U.S. officials July 2010. 21 states joined the suit in July 2011.

-Note: Statements and actions by state executive officials are listed for background information only. This report does not evaluate the role or positions of such officials.

Therefore it would be interesting to see if the States that actually oppose the health care law would in reality turn down the Federal government funds for Medicaid expansion and coverage within their individual states, especially considering that federal reimbursement for such expansion is much more generous than the average 57% Medicaid federal reimbursement prior to PPACA enactment. But some state officials were concerned that this federal reimbursement would not remain permanent. They worry that Congress might invariably decide to reduce the reimbursement rate. Hence their opposition to the Medicaid expansion mandate and subsequent suit against the health reform plan. Therefore the Supreme Court had to address 4 issues with regards to the suit against patient protection and Affordable care Act.

The 4 issues were as follows:

- Is the anti-Injunction Act applicable to the health care reform Act?
- Is the individual mandate within the constitutional authority of congress?
- If the Individual mandate is Unconstitutional, can it be severed from PPACA without nullifying the law?
- Is the Mandated Medicaid expansion Constitutional?[15]

The main issues of the suit challenging the constitutionality of the Affordable Care Act were succinctly summarized by National Conference of State Legislators (NCSl) as indicated in the chart below.

Table 4.2- Key Issues in NFIB v. Secretary Sebelius, Department of Health and Human Services

Issue	Federal Government Argued	State Plaintiffs Argued	U.S. Supreme Court Held
Is the challenge to the constitutionality of the individual mandate barred by the Tax Anti-Injunction Act? The Anti-Injunction Act (AIA) is a federal law that precludes, with certain exceptions, an individual from suing the federal government to stop a tax from being assessed or	The "penalty" for not purchasing health insurance is a "tax" because it is administered by the Internal Revenue Service. Under the Anti-Injunction Act, a tax may only be challenged after it has been assessed. The individual mandate is barred from the court's review until it becomes effective	The Anti-Injunction Act does not bar challenges to the individual mandate because individuals who do not purchase insurance must pay a "penalty" not a "tax." The goal of the "penalty" is to encourage individuals to purchase insurance, not to raise revenue.	The Anti-Injunction Act does not apply as a procedural bar to this case.

collected. This issue turns on whether the penalty for failure to purchase health insurance under the ACA is a tax under the AIA and subsequently barred from court review until the mandate becomes effective in 2014 and a penalty is assessed for failure to purchase qualified coverage is assessed in 2015?[1]	in 2014, a penalty is assessed for failure to purchase qualified coverage and the assessed penalty is challenged. This would likely occur when the individual files a 2014 tax return.		
Does the individual mandate exceed Congress' powers under the Commerce Clause of the U.S. Constitution? The Commerce Clause gives broad authority to the Congress on matters of interstate commerce and foreign trade.	Congress may require Americans to purchase health insurance pursuant to its constitutional authority to regulate commerce among the states. The individual mandate is a tool to help decrease cost shifting to individuals within the healthcare market.	The Mandate is unconstitutional because Congress lacks power to compel citizens to become active participants in a private market. The Commerce Clause grants Congress the authority to regulate "activity" within the commercial market; "inactivity" is outside of congressional control.	The court upheld the individual mandate as constitutional under Congress' Article 1 taxing power.
If the individual mandate is found to be unconstitutional, can other provisions of the ACA be saved? Does the lack of a	If the individual mandate is struck down, only two provisions of the law should not survive. The provision which pre-	The individual mandate is so "inextricably intertwined" with the other provisions of the law, that if it is ruled	The individual mandate was upheld.

severability clause in the ACA require the whole Act to fall if any provision is found to be unconstitutional? The ACA, unlike many acts, does not have a severability clause, which requires that if any provision is struck from the law, unrelated provisions remain in effect.	vents insurance companies from: (1) refusing coverage to individuals with pre-existing conditions; and (2) charging higher premiums based on a parson's medical history. The remainder of the law should stand because the other provisions are unrelated to the mandate.	unconstitutional, the entire law must fall due to the lack of a severability clause in the ACA.	
Did Congress unconstitutionally coerce the states into agreeing to substantially expand Medicaid by threatening to withhold states' federal Medicaid funding? At what point do grant conditions imposed on states by the federal government cross the line or, in the case of Medicaid, involve such a large part of a state's economy that participation in the program and the associated conditions are no longer voluntary.	Congress has the authority to attach conditions on the receipt of federal funds pursuant to its grant of power under the Spending Clause of the Constitution. The Supreme Court has never ruled any such condition coercive.	The Medicaid expansion is coercive. Medicaid funding has become so important to states that they must participate in the program and thus comply with the federal requirements. There must be some limit to the congressional regulation of states in this manner.	The court upheld the Medicaid expansion, but makes it a voluntary provision as opposed to a mandatory provision. The court would not permit HHS to penalize states by withholding all Medicaid funding for choosing not to participate in the expansion.

[1] Both the state plaintiffs and the federal government argued that the Tax Anti Injunc-
tion Act does not apply to the ACA's penalty. Source: NCSL, July 24, 2012[16]

Thus the main questions or issues that the Supreme Court had to address as mentioned earlier with the health care law challenge were the following: Can the suit
be brought to bear? Is the Patient Protection and Affordable Health Care Act
constitutional? Specifically is the individual mandate constitutional? Also is the
individual mandate severable from the health care Act. That is can the health
care Act survive if the individual mandate was declared unconstitutional? There
are two main analyses that can be utilized to answer the question regarding the
constitutionality of the health care law's individual mandate requirement.

One analysis could focus on whether the individual mandate is a proper
exercise of Congress's powers to regulate interstate commerce. Thus the question that would beg to be asked is whether the Interstate Commerce Act allows
the federal government to compel individuals to buy health care insurance which
they may not want to buy, when their non-purchase of the aforementioned health
insurance might harm others? It is important to note here, as mentioned earlier
that cost shifting will occur with private pay as well as other insured patients and
taxpayers eventually being on the hook for uncompensated hospital emergency
care expenses, if an uninsured person gets very sick and has to utilize hospital
emergency room care.

This brings up the issue of limiting principle. Limiting principle is the concept or idea of curtailing the power of congress to mandate individuals to buy
goods or services, in this instance, health care insurance. Under limiting principle, when the Supreme Court reviews a new application of Congressional application of a constitutional principle, they usually want an articulation of the limits
to such application of that principle.[17] So when a new congressional statue is
challenged constitutionally in court, the Supreme Court usually wants to know,
the boundaries of such congressional law. Thus, Congress cannot mandate individuals to buy goods or services except if there are limiting principles to such a
mandate. So if the Supreme Court cannot find a limiting principle to the health
care law's individual mandate requirement, then the individual mandate would
be deemed unconstitutional. On the other hand if the justices determine that
there is a limiting principle to the individual mandate then the mandate could
possibly pass muster. Therefore in order for the Supreme Court to find the individual mandate constitutional, the government has to show conclusively that
there are specific instances where government cannot compel people to buy
products and that such instances are specifically different from the individual
mandate. This is very important, because if congress can mandate people to purchase health insurance, what is to stop them from requiring people to buy other
products. Thus, the concept of limiting principle is to ensure that congressional
powers do not go unchecked. The limiting principle argument can be analyzed
though the scope of Adverse selection, Interstate Externalities principle, and
finally the taxation principle.

Adverse Selection

As interpreted by the Supreme Court, activities that can significantly affect commerce can be regulated by Congress. That means that Congress can, under the auspices of the necessary and proper clause, mandate individuals to engage in commercial activity, when needed to prevent adverse selection problems created by Congress's regulation of commerce. But if adverse selection is not an issue then Congress cannot compel commerce. The limiting principle can apply with regards to say for instance the government requiring people to buy broccoli or apples. Government does not have the right to do so. Thus if congress were to mandate that people should buy tomatoes, the Supreme Court will find that mandate unconstitutional. This is because if people do not choose to buy tomatoes which are healthy and good for them at the store, the tomatoes market would not collapse. There would be some individuals that would choose to buy tomatoes; likewise individuals can survive without ever buying tomatoes. A person can live to a ripe old age without ever wanting, needing or buying tomatoes.

But health care insurance is not the same as broccoli. Everybody at some point or time in their life will need health care. Usually if they have health care insurance, the health care services that they will need one day or the other would be mostly covered by their health insurance plans. But if individuals do not have health care insurance and they get sick, or need care, they will still need to be treated in emergency cases. For example if someone falls and breaks a leg or have a heart attack. The individual will need to be taken to the hospital. Now under the USA law EMTALA as mentioned previously, nobody can be turned away from the hospital for emergency health services, regardless of if they have insurance or not. They have to be stabilized at the hospital, that is, the health emergency episode has to be over or stabilized prior to the hospital releasing the individual. Now if they happened to be uninsured and as such could not pay for their physician and hospital emergency services, the uncompensated costs of their emergency health care services are going to be passed on to other consumers in the form of taxes that hospitals and providers charge to recoup the cost of uncompensated care. These taxes are likewise spread over the charges submitted by the providers to insurance companies, with the attendant eventual result that insurance premiums increase. Thus the effects of those individuals refusing to purchase health insurance and eventually utilizing medical health care which they could not pay for would be felt by individuals that actually purchase health care insurance. Under Congressional, Commerce Clause powers, Congress can compel people to purchase a good or service when, if market failure would occur otherwise. That is, if the market would collapse as a result of people's refusal to participate within the market, especially when they will definitely need the good or service and then would otherwise transfer the cost of using the service to the rest of the citizens.

The insurance companies likewise operate on the concept of a risk pool to spread the risk of its participants. If healthy individuals choose not to buy insurance and wait till they are sick to buy health insurance then the health insurance market would collapse, because the system would not be able to handle, the excessive amount of payout to the health care providers of their sick or unhealthy participants or enrollees. Therefore, in order for the concept of health insurance to work and for the health insurance industry to have a viable market, there needs to be a spread of healthy and sick people within the plan. So individuals opting out of health insurance plans have far reaching adverse consequences on the health insurance market.[18] According to Ezekiel Emanuel, "Voluntary health insurance exchanges piloted in several states without mandates all failed because healthy people opted out. Those who are relatively healthy figure the cost of insurance is too high, that they are subsidizing insurance premiums for sicker people and they probably (it is a risk) won't need the insurance because they are healthy. When some healthy people stop buying coverage, the premium goes up for the remaining slightly sicker people. Then, as premiums go up, more and more healthy people drop out, creating an inevitable downward spiral. This is cost-shifting from the uninsured to the insured, and it is true not just in theory, but in practice. We have tried many such exchanges, and they have all failed. Only the Massachusetts exchange has worked because of its mandate requiring healthy, as well as sicker, people to buy insurance."[19] This quotation reinforces the notion that it is important to have a mix of healthy and sick people participating within the health insurance plan, otherwise it would not work, because health insurance plans could not financially afford to have only the sick enroll within their plans.

Hence the reason why Congress structured the health care reform plan such that a wide risk pool is created by mandating individuals who do not have insurance either from their employers, Medicaid, Medicare or otherwise, to buy coverage through health Insurance exchanges. This reduces adverse selection.

The Interstate Externalities Principle

According to Econsterms, externality is defined as, "An effect of a purchase or use decision by one set of parties on others who did not have a choice and whose interests were not taken into account."[20] So when this definition is applied to the concept of interstate Externalities Principles or Interstate Spill Over Effect, it simply means that the actions or non-actions of group A individuals had subsequent (usually adverse) effects on another set of group B individuals within another state, whereby group B did not have any say or control over the actions/non-actions of group A. As such the interests of group B were not taken into consideration by group A during their actions or non-actions. Simply put, group B individuals in a different state were adversely affected by what group A did or did not do. Health care is a unique case that can cause interstate spill over costs, whereby some states bear the costs that should properly be borne by other states.[21] For instance with regards to health insurance, if certain states have individual mandates and assured coverage or very generous medical insurance coverage regardless of preexisting conditions, sicker people or uninsurable very sick people would tend to move to those states with individual mandate such that they could have health insurance, and in the process driving up premiums and health care costs there, thus creating an interstate externality in the process.

The Taxation Principle

The argument can properly be made that the individual health insurance mandate penalty is a tax. Congress has the power to impose taxes based on general welfare. The mandate penalty is an amendment to the Internal Revenue Code, and it is calculated based on a percentage of adjusted gross income or a fixed amount, whichever is larger. Starting in 2014, it will be collected on your form 1040 just like your other taxes. The issue with the health care law mandate is whether Congress has the power to regulate and tax a citizen for not participating in interstate commerce.

According to Chief Justice Roberts writing for the majority opinion, with respect to congressional power to regulate commerce, the individual mandate cannot be sustained. This is because Congress has the power to regulate what people do, but the constitution cannot be interpreted to give congress the power to regulate what people do not do. Interpreting the constitution otherwise would open up "New and potentially vast domain to congressional authority."[22] Accordingly, his opinion was that the framers of the Constitution gave congress the power to regulate commerce not to compel it. [23]

Likewise, the individual mandate cannot be sustained under the necessary and proper clause of PPACA. This is because the Supreme Court's precedents for upholding the clause involved cases whereby there was exercise of authority that stemmed from and in application of a granted power. For example, in the case of United States v Comstock 560, a case that was decided by the Supreme Court in 2010, the high court upheld the necessary and proper clause in that case, and ruled that the clause grants congress the authority necessary to require civil commitment of individuals that were already in federal custody. Accordingly, the authority to do so, stemmed from the implied power to punish individuals that break the law. In that case, Graydon Comstock was charged and sentenced to 37 months incarceration for receiving child pornography. Six days prior to the completion of his sentence, Attorney General Alberto Gonzales certified to a federal district Judge that Comstock was a sexually dangerous person and had to be civilly committed. When such a certification is filed, according to the Adam Walsh Child Protection and Safety Act of 2006,[24] the individual is automatically precluded from being released from prison. This provides the government the opportunity to have a hearing to prove its claims through psychiatric evidence or otherwise.[25] Comstock brought a suit claiming that the federal government did not have the right to certify him to be civilly committed. He contended that it was outside the enumerated powers granted by the Constitution to congress. The Supreme Court held that the necessary and proper clause, grants Congress the authority necessary to require civil commitment of individuals that were already in federal custody.[26] Thus in this case, the excise of the Adam Walsh Child Protection and Safety Act of 2006, stemmed from the implied power to punish individuals that break the law and there is further inference of the power to imprison or commit, in application of the necessary and proper cause.

The Supreme Court on the other hand, opinioned that the individual mandate under the health reform law, grants Congress the power to "Create the necessary predicate to the exercise of an enumerated power and draw within its regulatory scope those who would otherwise be outside of it. Even if the individual mandate is "necessary" to the Affordable Care Act's other reforms, such an expansion of federal power are not a "proper" means for making those reforms effective."[27] Therefore the court believed that the federal government was utilizing the individual mandate to bring in within its regulatory powers, people that would normally have been outside its powers, in this case the individuals that choose not to buy health insurance, whom would not normally be considered economic players within interstate commerce.

But the Court went on further to determine that the individual mandate can be upheld when construed as a tax despite the fact that the reform law refers to it as a penalty. Therefore the court utilized a functional approach when it reasoned that the substance of the mandate not the exact wording holds the key to determination of whether the fines for not purchasing health care insurance could be construed as a tax. Thus, under the functional approach, the court reasoned that the shared responsibility fines of the individual mandate fell within the constructs of a tax. Especially considering the fact that the penalty is not so high that individuals will have no choice but to buy health insurance and the penalty does not attach any unlawful consequences to non-purchase of health insurance, except to require an IRS payment. Thus one can construe the penalty of the individual mandate, simply as an imposition of a tax on those who do not have health insurance.[28] And if that is the case then the penalty that attaches to the individual mandate requirement is constitutional, under the taxation doctrine.

The whole premise of the health care Act is that Congress has the power to enact such a law because of the powers vested onto Congress by the Commerce Clause. According to Article I, Section 8, Clause 3 of the Constitution, "The Congress shall have Power ...To regulate Commerce with foreign Nations, and among the several states." This is known as the Commerce Clause. The Supreme Court has interpreted this portion of the constitution to mean that Congress has the power to oversee any activity that has commercial impact across state lines. As such the Commerce clause have been utilized extensively by congress as a means of welding control over a lot of activities that can be minimally considered to have an impingement on interstate commerce. A somewhat recent Supreme Court precedent with regards to congressional reach via the interstate commence Act is the Supreme Court's decision in Gonzales v. Raich, (2005).[29] The High Court ruled that, although Ms. Raich, was using home grown marijuana on doctors' orders, the production of the crop (in this case marijuana) has a substantial effect on the national demand and supply of marijuana. According to the court, "The proper test of the reaches of Congress' power is not whether the product is meant to move in commerce but whether its production and use has a "substantial economic effect on interstate commerce."[30] Therefore, regardless of the fact that Ms. Raich's use was intrastate and was likewise under state sanctioned medical orders, Congress could still regulate personal and intrastate use of products or goods so long as that use has a potential for significant fiscal effect on interstate commerce.

The substantial effects test had an impact on the Supreme Court ruling with regards to the constitutionality of PPACA. According to the Supreme Court, Congress has the power to regulate interstate Commerce and accordingly health insurance which would be considered interstate commerce. Therefore, reasoned the Supreme Court, PPACA was within the constitutional jurisdiction of Congress. This is especially true since health insurance and health care costs can have a substantial economic effect on interstate commerce.

Thus on June 28th 2012, the Supreme Court ruled that the suit against the health reform Act was not barred from proceeding by the Anti-Injunction Act. The Anti-Injunction Act (AIA) usually bars or prevents, an individual or entity from suing to stop the federal government from assessing or collecting a tax. In the case of the suit against PPACA, the issue is whether the penalty assessed under the health reform Act for failure to purchase health insurance constitutes a tax under AIA and as such precluded from court review until the effective date of the mandate in 2014, when the attendant penalty is assessed in 2015 for nonpurchase of health insurance.[31] Usually under the Anti-Injunction Act the law could not be challenged until the penalty has been meted out, then it could be challenged. At the same time that the Supreme Court ruled that AIA did not bar the lawsuit against PPACA from proceeding, it likewise ruled that the Individual Mandate was Constitutional under Article 1 Taxing powers. As such, the issue of severability did not come into play, since the individual mandate was ruled to be constitutional and thus the question did not arise regarding if it could be severed from the body of the health reform law without nullifying the whole law. The Supreme Court also ruled that the Patient Protection and Affordable Care Act was constitutional and as such upheld the provisions of the health reform act, with one exception. The high Court placed limitation on the penalties that would have accrued to the states if they would not expand their Medicaid rolls. Therefore the Supreme Court upheld the Medicaid expansion provision of the act, but only as a voluntary provision for the states in lieu of a mandatory requirement. That means that the states could choose to opt out of the Medicaid expansion requirement, but the department of Health and Human Services under the auspices of the federal government could not penalize any state that chose not to expand their Medicaid rolls, by withholding all of their original federal Medicaid funding, as was initially stipulated within the health reform Act.

Some of the other health insurance alternatives to PPACA that had been mentioned within public media are the single payer health care system and the public option health care system. The single payer system would have been similar to the health care system in Canada whereby the government collects all the revenues, usually in the form of taxes, to finance the universal health care system and they likewise pay out money for medical services provided. The money could be paid to private medical providers or the government could provide the medical services. Medicare is an example of such a system whereby the government collects the fees through payroll taxes in the form of Federal Insurance Contributions Act (FICA) and then pays out or covers 80% of the cost of health services provided usually by private health care providers to seniors over the age of 65 years old. Individual or private gap insurance covers the balance or 20% of cost of the senior's medical services.[32] If USA were to have a single payer system, it would most likely be similar to Medicare but with no age restriction. Countries such as Canada and Sweden have such a system. It should be contrasted with the system in United Kingdom, which some consider socialized medicine, whereby the government owns the hospitals and the doctors, nurses and other employees of the hospitals are considered government workers.

The single payer system most likely, would have been found constitutional by the Supreme Court under the tax and spend powers of congress. This is because, according to Article 1, Section 8, Clause 1 of the Constitution states: "The Congress shall have the Power to lay and collect taxes...for the general welfare."[33] As such, the premiums collected for health care system under the single payer system would be within the constraints of the aforementioned constitutional powers, because the payment for such health insurance would clearly fall under the concept of a tax.

The public health option, on the other hand was considered by democrats prior to enactment of PPACA, but it was dropped during congressional negotiations, when it seemed unlikely that it would garner enough support for the health care reform bill to pass. Public option is a proposed health care system whereby individuals and businesses have a choice of choosing between government provided health insurance (similar to Medicare) versus private health insurance, which provided the bulk of health insurance policies prior to PPACA. So it can be considered a type of hybrid system that meshes both aspects of the single payer system like Medicare and private health insurance. Thus it is feasible that under a public option heath care plan, individuals could still keep their private insurance if they so choose, while uninsured or underinsured individuals would go with the public option. Proponents believe that this would provide needed competition within the health care market place between government provided health insurance versus private health insurance. According to an October 2009, poll by Washington post, "If a public plan were run by the states and available only to those who lack affordable private options, support for it jumps to 76 percent. Under those circumstances, even a majority of Republicans, 56 percent, would be in favor of it, about double their level of support without such a limitation."[34] Invariably the public option did not make it to the final health care reform bill that was signed by President Obama. But the public option would also most likely have been found constitutional by the Supreme Court because of the constitutional stipulation that Congress has the power to collect and lay taxes. In this instance there would be a health care premiums "tax" assessed for the public option coverage.

Despite the lawsuit and eventual subsequent decision by the Supreme Court, several states had already begun the effort of ensuring compliance with the mandates of the Health reform Act, prior to the Supreme Court's ruling on the case on June 28, 2012. The Act required implementation timetables for uniform, 50 state requirements and options that would enhance existing state regulation of insurance policies. Thus the states would have to address issues regarding uniform price insurance coverage for individuals with pre-existing conditions, family coverage that would likewise cover dependents up to the age of 26, premium rates reviews etc. Thus far an appreciable number of states have made progress towards such uniform requirements. Such compliance efforts were started as early as 2010 by some of the states, and by 2011, quite a few states had enacted laws that would bring them in compliance with the mandates of PPACA. The information from the table below is from the National Conference of State Legislators

Table 4.3- The States That Enacted Laws in 2011 and the Nature of the Laws Enacted.

Policy in 2011 or 2012 Enacted State Law	States- 2011	# of States	States- 2012	# of States
Adult dependents- requiring family policies to allow coverage for adult dependents up to age 26 [NCSL Fact Sheet]	Delaware, Kentucky, Minnesota, South Dakota, Virginia	5		
Any willing provider- certain providers or facilities must be able to participate in health insurance benefit delivery	North Dakota	1	Oregon	1
Child- only health policies to be offered by health insurers serving the individual market	Arkansas, Colorado, Washington	3	Georgia	1
Confidentiality protection for providers	Tennessee	1		
Consumer protection coverage for pre-existing conditions [NCSL Report]	Hawaii, Indiana, Maryland, Oklahoma	4		
External Review or independent appeal of coverage denials for consumers [NCSL Report]	Hawaii, Iowa, Nevada, North Dakota, Ohio, Oregon, Virginia	7	Delaware, Washington	2

General insurance re-forms, requiring coordination with ACA- Broad implementation of ACA insurance provisions, 2011-2013	California, Indiana, Illinois, Maine, Michigan, Minnesota, New Hampshire, New York, North Carolina, Oregon, Pennsylvania, Utah, Vermont	13	Connecticut, Maine, Maryland, Rhode Island, South Dakota, Vermont, Washington	7
Health/ Wellness Program coverage within health policies	Tennessee	1		
High Risk Pools: the federal "pre-existing Conditions Insurance Program" [NCSL Report]	Nebraska, Oregon, South Dakota	3	Illinois, Kansas, Washington	3
HSA'S/High deductible health policies integrated with ACA	Wisconsin	1		
Mandates defining or requiring health insurance or requiring health insurance coverage or services [examples; additional mandate laws]	Arkansas, California, Colorado, Louisiana, Montana, Rhode Island, West Virginia	7	Louisiana, Utah, West Virginia	3
Additional mandate laws, not referencing ACA. A full list of mandate laws is in Table 3.	Arkansas, California, Colorado, Connecticut, Delaware, Georgia, Indiana, Illinois, Louisiana, Maryland, Montana, New Hampshire, New Jersey, New Mexico, New York, Oregon, Rhode Island, Tennessee, Texas, Vermont, Virginia, Washington, West Virginia	23		13
Medical Loss Ratios (MLR) defining minimum expenditures of health services [NCSL Report]	Connecticut, Georgia, Idaho, Maine	4	Maryland, Nebraska	2
Premium Rate Review, coordinating state and federal requirements	Maine, New Mexico, North Carolina, North Dakota, South Dakota, Tennessee, Ver-	8	Vermont	1

[NCSL Report]	mont, Washington			
Single payer universal coverage as an alternative to ACA provisions	Illinois, Vermont	2		
Small employer health coverage	Arizona, Missouri	2	Delaware, Vermont	2
State employee health plans coordinated with ACA	Connecticut, Idaho, Massachusetts, Nevada, Wisconsin, Utah	6	Georgia, Utah	2
Out-of-State policies available for in-state sale [NCSL Report]	Georgia, Maine	2	Kentucky	1
Other	Delaware, Hawaii, Massachusetts, Mississippi, Oklahoma	5	Arizona, Illinois, Hawaii, Maine, New Jersey, Rhode Island, Virginia Washington	8

Source: National Conference of State Legislators (NCSL), July 12 2012.[35]

---

1. Medicaid is the largest health insurance program for both indigent and disabled individuals. Medicaid was enacted under Title XIX of the Social Security Act, in 1964. It is a joint state and federal government assisted health-insurance program for the poor. The states determine the eligibility criteria for enrolling its indigent uninsured population within their Medicaid programs and the federal government reimburses them at a rate of 57% of their state funding for Medicaid.
2. Certain legal immigrants may also qualify.
3. What is Medicare? (n.d.). Retrieved July 25, 2012, from Centers for Medicare and Medicaid Services: http://www.medicare.gov/publications/pubs/pdf/11306.pdf.
4. Goodwin, L., & Wilson, C. (2012, June 29). Map: Where ObamaCare Would Expand Medicaid Most. Retrieved July 13, 2012, from Yahoo News: http://news.yahoo.com/blogs/ticket/map-where-ObamaCare-expand-medicaid-most-175400889.html
5. Usually, Health insurance companies can charge women more for coverage. They can also decide not to extend health insurance coverage to individuals with preexisting conditions. In the instances that they cover them, it I usually at a much higher rate than the norm.
6. Elmendorf, D. W. (2011, March 30). CBO's Analysis of the Major Health Care Legislation Enacted in March 2012. Retrieved July 13, 2012, from CBO: http://www.cbo.gov/sites/default/files/cbofiles/ftpdocs/121xx/doc12119/03-30-healthcarelegislation.pdf
7. CBO's 2011 Long-term Budget Outlook. (2011, June 22). Retrieved July 13, 2012, from CBO: http://cbo.gov/publication/41486
8. Elmendorf
9. Remarks by the President on Supreme Court Ruling on the Affordable Care Act. (2012, June 28). Retrieved July 14, 2012, from The White House:

http://www.whitehouse.gov/the-press-office/2012/06/28/remarks-president-supreme-court-ruling-affordable-care-act
10. Medicaid. (2012). Retrieved July 14, 2012, from The New York Times:http://topics.nytimes.com/top/news/health/diseasesconditionsandhealthtopics/medicaid/index.html
11. It is important to note that the federal government pays on average about 57% of all the states Medicaid costs. Usually the federal government pays about 50 percent of the costs in higher-income states like Massachusetts and more, about 70 percent in lower-income states like Mississippi.
12. Goodwin and Wilson
13. Ibid
14. Ibid
15. U.S. Supreme Court and the Federal Health Law. (2012, July 24). Retrieved August 5, 2012, from National Conference of State Legislators: http://www.ncsl.org/issues-research/health/us-supreme-court-and-the-federal-health-law.aspx
16. Ibid
17. Joyner, J. (2012, March 27). ObamaCare Mandate Limiting Principle. Retrieved July 21, 2012, from Outside the Beltway: http://www.outsidethebeltway.com/ObamaCare-mandate-limiting-principle/
18. Emanuel, E. (n.d.). Here's Why Health Insurance is Not Like Broccoli. Retrieved July 19, 2012, from http://blogs.reuters.com/great-debate/2012/03/29/heres-why-health-insurance-is-not-like-broccoli/.
19. Ibid
20 . Definition of Externality. (n.d.). Retrieved from Econterms: http://economics.about.com/cs/economicsglossary/g/externality.htm.
21. Ahmar, A. R. (n.d.). How to Defend ObamaCare. Retrieved July 21, 2012, from Slate:http://www.slate.com/articles/news_and_politics/jurisprudence/2012/03/supreme_court_and_ObamaCare_what_donald_verrilli_should_have_said_to_the_court_s_conservative_justices_.html
22. National Federation of Independent Business, et al. v. Sebelius Secretary of Health and Human Services, et al. (2012, June 28). Retrieved July 20, 2012, from http://www.supremecourt.gov/opinions/11pdf/11-393c3a2.pdf
23. Ibid.
24. Adam Walsh Child Protection and Safety Act of 2006, otherwise known as the Sex Offender Registration and Notification Act (SORNA), was signed into law on July 27, 2006, by then President George W Bush. It was named for a young USA boy named Adam Walsh, who was kidnapped from a Florida shopping mall in 1981 and was later found murdered. The Act created a sex offender registry, specifies sex offender registration requirements for convicted sex offenders, and makes it harder for predators to reach children on the Internet. The Act is likewise intended to help prevent child abuse by creating a National Child Abuse Registry. It also requires that adoptive and foster parents be subjected to background checks prior to assuming custody of a child and has provisions for civil commitment of sexually dangerous persons.
25. United States v. Comstock et al. (2010, May 17). Retrieved July 22, 2012, from http://www.supremecourt.gov/opinions/09pdf/08-1224.pdf
26. Ibid
27. National Federation of Independent Business, et al. v. Sebelius Secretary of Health and Human Services, et al.
28. Ibid

29. Under California's Compassionate Use Act, private individuals could grow and culti- vate marijuana for their personal and medical use. Angel Raich and Diane Monson were two Californians that grew marijuana for their medical personal use. Under the Federal Controlled Substance Act (CSA), their house was raided by federal agents, who then destroyed and seized their medical cannabis plant. The two sued to preclude enforcement of the CSA, claiming that it was an unlawful application of the interstate commerce Act for federal agents to apply CSA, a federal law to their situation. Accordingly, this was especially true, since they were growing the cannabis for non-commercial intrastate per- sonal medical consumption. The plaintiffs lost their case and they appealed. The US court of Appeals for the 9th circuit, ruled in their favor thus enjoining application of CSA to their situation. The Government petitioned the Supreme Court for Certiorari. The Su- preme court reversed the decision of the appellate court opining that although the behav- ior was intrastate and involved marijuana for personal use, nonetheless the commerce clause , gives Congress the power to regulate solely personal and intrastate activity. (GONZALES V. RAICH (03-1454) 545 U.S. 1 (2005) 352 F.3d 1222)
30. Gonzales v. Raich: Implications For Public Health Policy. (2005). Public Health Representative, 680-682.
31. U.S. Supreme Court and the Federal Health Law
32 . Is Health Care Reform Constitutional? (n.d.). Retrieved July 17, 2012, from Constitutionland Development Corporation: http://www.constitutionland.com/ Health_care_Reform.html
33. Ibid
34. Balz, D., & Cohen, J. (2009, October 20). Most Support Public Option for Health Insurance, Poll finds. Retrieved July 17, 2012, from Washington Post: http://www.washingtonpost.com/wpdyn/content/article/2009/10/19/AR2009101902451.h tml
35. Health Insurance Reform Enacted State Laws Related to the Affordable Health Care Act. (2011 and 2012). Retrieved July 27, 2012, from National Conference of State Legislators: http://www.ncsl.org/issues-research/health/2012-health-insurance-reform- state-laws.aspx

Chapter 5

Main Components of the Patient Protection and Affordable Care Act

The Patient Protection and Affordable Health Care Act was signed into law on March 23rd 2010 alongside with the corresponding Health Care and Education Reconciliation Act on March 30th 2010, with the broad goals of expanding health insurance to uninsured individuals. As such the key indices for PPACA are as follows:

Stronger Consumer Rights and Protections:
Prior to enactment of Patient Protection and Affordable Care Act, insurance companies had a lot of leeway in whom they would decide to insure and whom they would not insure. They could cancel your health insurance policy on the pretext that there was a mistake in your original insurance application. They could also put a lifetime limit on the cost of care that they would provide to an individual, or deny a child health child insurance simply because the child has a preexisting condition such as asthma or sickle cell anemia. But the health reform act brought into play stronger consumer rights and protections. Some of these consumer rights and protections are discussed below.

End to Limits on Care:
The new health care reform plan incorporates a patient bill of rights that guarantees several protections to patients that were not formerly available prior to enactment of the Act. For instance prior to PPACA, health insurance companies could set an annual or lifetime dollar limit on the cost of coverage that they would provide a patient. Thus once the lifetime limit is reached, the health insurance company does not need to pay anymore for that particular patient's health care bills. Therefore prior to PPACA, if a patient had several expensive surgeries and treatments for cancer and the patient happened to be involved in an auto accident that required extensive and very expensive treatment and rehabilitation, the patient could max out their lifetime dollar limit of coverage which could result in the health insurance company denying further coverage of the

required medical treatment. This would leave the patient with either stopping the needed treatment or trying to find a means of paying for the treatment out of pocket. This is especially true for individuals that might need a series of very expensive treatment, such as care after serious accident and injury, repeated heart surgeries, reoccurring cancer treatments etc. The new health care law precludes insurance companies from setting lifetime dollar limits on the cost of essential care for their insured members, and starting from 2014, there would be no more annual limits on coverage for essential care.

End to Coverage Cancellations:
The Health Care Act precludes health insurance companies from dropping an insured patient from their policy, when the patient is sick, simply because they happened to notice a mistake within the patient's insurance application. [1] The insurance companies would sometimes use this tactic to cancel the insurance of individuals they deem high use or high utilization. As such the insurance company would carefully look over an insured individual's application, in the instances that the insured is requiring a lot of treatments. They thus can utilize this option as a loophole for cancelling the insurance policy of members that they think are utilizing too much health care services and as such are costing them a lot of money in paying for insured care.

 End to pre-existing Condition Discrimination:
Prior to enactment of the Health Care Act, health insurance companies could decide not to provide coverage for individuals with preexisting conditions such as diabetes, high blood pressure, heart failure, cancer etc. A preexisting condition means that the disease or disability was present prior to the participant enrolling in a health care plan. This was especially true of children with conditions such as asthma, diabetes etc. The enactment of the law ensured that upon implementation of PPACA, children younger than age 19, with preexisting conditions would no longer be denied health insurance. This rule is applicable to all individual health insurance plans as well as all job related health plans that were issued after March, 2010. This rule affects a health insurance plan that starts a policy or plan year on or after September 23, 2010. [2] This provision would be extended to adults starting from 2014, when no American would be denied health care coverage because of a preexisting condition. It is important to note that this provision does not apply to Grandfathered [3] Individual health insurance policies. Grandfathered health plans are subject only to a few requirements under PPACA with differing effective dates. Some of the requirements include the mandate for development of uniform explanation of benefits. Such plans must also report financial information and Medical Loss Ratios to the Secretary of Health and Human Services. If the plans do not meet specified medical loss ratios they must offer premium rebates to enrollees starting no later than January 1, 2011. [4] Then from September 23, 2010, such grandfathered plans, must abolish lifetime limits on essential health coverage, they must also abolish health coverage rescission or cancellation and they must extend coverage to enrollee's de-

pendents until they are 26 years old. A health plan rescission refers to when the insurance carrier that issued the health policy plan rescinds or cancels the policy of an enrollee and then treats the enrollee as if he/she was never enrolled in the plan such that the enrollee is left without any health insurance coverage and is responsible for all health costs incurred while previously covered.[5] It must be clarified that coverage for a dependent on a grandfathered plan prior to 2014, was only possible if such dependent was not eligible for employment based health benefits. [6]

More Affordable Coverage

The health reform law is predicated on the assumption that it would expand coverage while bringing down costs of health insurance. It is supposed to do this by adhering to specific provisions of the health care law.

Value for your Premium Dollar:
PPACA has an 80/20 rule that went into effect summer of 2012. The 80/20 rule basically says that if insurance companies spend less than 80 percent of enrollee's monthly/yearly premium dollars on medical care and quality improvements, in lieu of overhead, bonuses for executives and advertising, they will have to provide the insurance purchaser a rebate.

Justify Rate Increases:
The law requires for the first time in the history of health insurance in the USA, that health insurance companies within every state of the union must publicly justify the reason for any stipulated rate increase above 10 percent. This makes it harder for insurance companies to arbitrarily raise health insurance premiums, since they would have to let the public know the reasons why the premium rates would increase over 10 percent. It must be noted that this does not apply to smaller insurance premium increases that are less than 10 percent. Thus insurance companies could foreseeably have premium increases of for example nine percent without having to justify such an increase.

Tax Credits for Small Businesses:
Usually in the past, small businesses have paid higher insurance premiums than larger businesses. Sometimes up to 18 percent more than larger employers. This was because small businesses, unlike large businesses and companies, do not have the large participant mixture that makes it possible for risk to be spread amongst a large pool of insured individuals. Since they do not have a large participant mixture their premiums tend to be higher so as to offset the higher associated risk inherent with providing coverage for a smaller pool of people. The health care reform law provides tax credit for about 360,000 estimated small businesses, which in turn will benefit the about 2 million workers who get their insurance from such small businesses.[7]

Better Access to Health Care:
PPACA was enacted with the idea that the reform plan will also provide better access to care for insured individuals. The basis is that participants would have more health insurance companies to choose from especially considering that participants would no longer be limited by preexisting conditions, lifetime benefit caps etc. and likewise would have more opportunities to receive needed care.

The plan would do that by incorporating the following:

Free Prevention Benefits:
Since the inception of the reform plan, health insurers must now cover recommended preventive services such as diabetes, cancer, cholesterol, blood pressure screenings etc. without requiring additional cost sharing from the patient such as copays or deductibles. Since it has been in effect, about 54 million Americans with private health insurance coverage have gotten expanded preventive services coverage.[8]

Health insurance Coverage for Young Adults:
Prior to enactment of PPACA, there were Approximately 13 million or 30 percent of young Americans without health insurance. These demographics were between the ages of 19 and 29.[9] Prior to the enactment of the new health care law, young adults could not stay on their parents insurance plans once they were adults. The age limits and stipulations differed from state to state, but in Tennessee under Tennessee Code Ann. § 56-7-2302 children up to age 24 that were unmarried and financially dependent on their parents, could stay on their parents' health insurance plan. Under the new law, most young adults up until the age of 26, who could not get coverage through their jobs, could stay on their parents' plans until age 26. This is irrespective of if they are in school, working, married, live with parent, or are not financially dependent on parent, provided that they are not eligible for group coverage through an employer. This does not mean that an insurer has to provide insurance singly to the dependent; it simply means that if the insurer offers the plan then it must extend it to the dependent of the insured. Under the issued regulations of the Act, even if the youth is eligible for a discount plan, he/she would still be covered under the parents plan.[10] This is applicable to all plans within the individual market as well as to employer plans that were created after March 23 2010. For grandfathered health insurance plans or plans that were in place prior to March 23, 2010, young adults could only qualify for dependent coverage if they are not eligible for an employment-based health insurance until 2014. Starting from 2014, you adults would then have the choice of staying on their parent's health plans; that means that instead of enrolling in their employer health plan, they could choose to stay on their parent's health plan until they are 26 years old, regardless of whether they are eligible for their own employer sponsored health insurance plan.[11] This law does

not require that a plan or issuer offer dependent coverage but that if such coverage is offered it must be extended to young adults up to age 26.[12]

Individual states within the nation could apply their individual state regulations with regards to extended coverage for dependent adults so long as such application does not preclude the mandates or application of PPACA. Prior to enactment of PPACA, about 37 different states of the union had already extended dependent coverage within their states, although each state's eligibility requirements can differ significantly from those of other states. About 30 states extended dependent coverage regardless of whether the dependent is a student or not. The majority of the states however mandate that in order to be eligible for extended dependent coverage, the dependent be unmarried and financially dependent on parents.[13]

According to data from National Conference of State legislatures, as of June 2010, prior to 23rd September of 2010, when the mandated extended dependent coverage as per PPACA was slated to go into effect, the following states had enacted the specific actions mentioned therein.

Table 5.1- State Laws with Regards to Dependent Children

State	Laws
Colorado	Colo. Rev. Stat. § 10-16-104.3 states that a child is considered a dependent for insurance purposes up to age 25 (even if they are not enrolled in an educational institution) as long as they are unmarried and are financially dependent or share the same permanent address as the insurance provider.
Connecticut	C.G.S.A. § 38a-497 requires that group comprehensive and health insurance policies extend coverage to unwed children until the age of 26 provided they remain residents of Connecticut or are full-time students.
Delaware	Del. Code Ann. Tit. 18, § 3354 requires insurance providers to cover policyholder's dependent children until age 24. Dependents must be unmarried and a resident of Delaware or, if living outside the state, a full-time students. Insurance companies may charge more for dependent coverage past age 18, but it may not exceed 102 percent of the policyholder's cost before the child turned 18.
Florida	Florida 627.6562 allows for dependent children up to 25, who live with their parent or are a student, and up to 30 years old, who are also unmarried and have no dependent child of their own, to remain on their parents' insurance.
Georgia	Ga. Code § 33-30-4 allows dependent children up to age

	25 who are enrolled as a full-time student at least five months during the year or are eligible to enroll but are prevented due to illness or injury to remain on their parents' insurance. Ga. Code § 33-24-28 requires that a health services plan or health insurer exempt dependent children incapable of self-sustaining employment due to disability from dependent age limits.
Idaho	Idaho Stat. § 41-2103 allows for any unmarried dependents to remain on their parents' health insurance until age 21; any full-time, unmarried student until age 25; or a dependent with a disability without regard to age.
Illinois	215 ILCS 5/356z.12 provides parents with the option of keeping unmarried dependents on their health care insurance up to age 26. Parents with dependents who are veterans can keep them on their plans up to age 30.
Indiana	IC 27-8-5-2, 28 and IC 27-13-7-3 require commercial health insurers and health maintenance organizations to cover children until age of 24 or without regard to age if they are incapable of self-sustaining employment due to disability.
Iowa	Iowa Code § 509.3 and Iowa Code § 514E.7 requires that health insurance providers continue to cover unmarried children under their parents' coverage provided that the child 1) is under the age of 25 and a current resident of Iowa, 2) is a full-time student, or 3) has a disability.
Kentucky	Ky. Rev. Stat. § 304.17A-256 allows parents to keep their unmarried children on their health plans until the age of 25. Parents may have to pay extra for their adult children.
Louisiana	La. Rev. Stat. Ann. § 22:1003 allows an unmarried, dependent child to remain on parent's insurance up to age 24 if they are a full-time student.
Maine	24-A MRSA § 2742-B requires individual and group health insurance policies to continue coverage for a dependent child up to 25 years of age if the child is dependent upon the policyholder and the child has no dependents of the his/her own.
Maryland	MD Code, Insurance § 15-418 requires that health insurance be extended to, at the request of the policy holder, unmarried dependents under the age of 25.
Massachusetts	Mass. Gen. Laws Ann. Ch. 175 § 108 allows dependents to stay on their parent's coverage for two years past the

	age of dependency or until age 26, whichever occurs first, or without regard to age if they are incapable of self-sustaining employment due to disability. Young adults ages 19-26 are eligible for lower-cost insurance coverage, tailored to meet their needs, offered through the Commonwealth Health Insurance Connector. Reform summary and fact sheet, PowerPoint presentation.
Minnesota	Minnesota Chapter 62E.02 Defines "dependent" as a spouse or unmarried child under age 25, or a dependent child of any age who is disabled.
Missouri	Mo. Rev. Stat. § 354-536 defines dependent as an unmarried child up to age 26. If a health maintenance organization plan provides that coverage of a dependent child terminates upon attainment of the limiting age for dependent children, such coverage shall continue while the child is and continues to be both incapable of self-sustaining employment by reason of mental or physical handicap and chiefly dependent upon the enrollee for support and maintenance.
Montana	MCA 33-22-140 provides insurance coverage under a parent's policy for unmarried children up to age 25.
Nevada	NRS 689C.055 allows an unmarried, dependent child who is a full-time student to remain on his or her parent's insurance up to age 24 if parent is covered by small group policy. NRS 689B.035 requires that dependents retain coverage beyond age of policy termination if they are incapable of self-sustaining employment due to disability.
New Hampshire	N.H. Rev. Stat § 420-B:8-aa defines dependent as those who are unmarried up to age 26 and either a full-time student or resident of New Hampshire for purposes of health insurance coverage. 2009 SB 115 allows those up to age 26 to buy-in to coverage through the state's CHIP program, Healthy Kids.
New Jersey	N.J.S.A. 17B:27-30.5 states that, at the option of the insured person, a dependent may be covered up to the age of 31, as long as they are unmarried and have no dependents of their own.
New Mexico	NM Stat. Ann. § 13-7-8 states that health insurance for dependents may not be terminated based on age up to

	age 25.
New York	2009 AB 9038 allows an unmarried child to remain on parent's insurance up to age 30 if they are a resident of New York.
North Dakota	N.D. Cent. Code § 26.1-36-22 allows an unmarried, dependent child to remain on parent's insurance up to age 22 if they live with parents. If they are a full-time student, they can remain on parent's insurance from age 22 up to age 26.
Ohio	Ohio Rev. Code § 1751.14, as amended by 2009 OH H 1 allows an unmarried, dependent child that is an Ohio resident or a full-time student to remain on parent's insurance up to age 28, or without regard to age if they are incapable of self-sustaining employment due to disability.
Oregon	O.R.S. § 735.720 defines dependent as an unmarried child up to 23, elderly parents and disabled adult children for the purpose of insurance coverage.
Pennsylvania	2009 SB 189 states that an unmarried child may remain on parent's insurance up to age 30 if they have no dependents and are residents of PA or are enrolled as full-time students. 51 Pa.C.S.A. § 7309 states that full-time students whose studies are interrupted by service in the reserves or the National Guard must be extended health care benefits as a dependent of their parent beyond the terminating age equal to the length of their deployment.
Rhode Island	R.I. Gen. Laws § 27-20-45 and Gen. Laws § 27-41-61 requires insurance plans which cover dependent children to cover unmarried dependent children until age 19 or, if a student, until age 25. If the dependent child is mentally or physically impaired, the plan must continue their coverage after the specified age.
South Carolina	S.C. Code Ann. § 38-71-1330 allows an unmarried, dependent child who is a full-time student to remain on parent's insurance up to age 22 if parent is covered by small group policy. S.C. Code Ann. § 38-71-350 requires that a dependent child who is not capable of self-sustaining employment be allowed to remain on his or her parent's insurance, without regard to age.
South Dakota	SD Codified Laws Ann. § 3-12A-1 states that any insur-

	ance provider offering benefits to a dependent may not terminate those benefits by reason of age before the dependent's 19th birthday. If the dependent is enrolled in an educational institution, they are not to be terminated until they reach age 24 and not terminated if unable to seek self-support due to disability. SD Codified Laws § 58-17-2.3 states that if the dependent remains a full-time student upon attaining age 24 but not exceeding age 29, the insurer shall provide for the continuation of coverage for that dependent at the insured's option.
Tennessee	Tennessee Code Ann. § 56-7-2302 allows for dependent coverage for children under their parents' health insurance plan up to age 24 provided the child is unmarried and financially dependent on the parents.
Texas	V.T.C.A. Insurance Code § 846.260 and V.T.C.A. Insurance Code § 1201.059 make dependent status available for an unmarried child up to age 25 for insurance purposes.
Utah	Utah Code Ann. tit. 31A § 22-610.5 requires that coverage for unmarried dependents continue up to age 26, regardless of whether or not the dependent is enrolled in higher education.
Virginia	Va. Code Ann. § 38.2-3525 makes dependent status available to any child up to age 19 or who is a dependent up to age 25 who resides with the parent or is a full-time student.
Washington	West's RCWA 48.44.215 states that, at the option of the insured person, an unmarried dependent may be covered up to age 25.
West Virginia	W. Va. Code § 33-16-1a defines dependent for health insurance coverage as a child or stepchild up to age 25.
Wisconsin	Wis. Stat. § 632.885 requires that coverage for unmarried dependents through a parent's insurance be offered up to age 27 if they are not offered insurance through an employer. Full-time students called to active duty in the armed forces can be covered beyond age 26 depending on various factors.
Wyoming	Wyo. Stat. § 26-19-302 states that if child is unmarried and a full-time student, they can remain on parent's insurance up to age 23 if parent is covered by small group policy.

Source: State Health Facts and NCSL, June 2010[14]

Coverage for Preexisting Conditions

Prior to enactment of PPACA, a great number of Americans were either locked or priced out of the health insurance market if they had a preexisting condition. That is because most insurance companies would either refuse to accept them as new participants within the insurance plan or they would charge them such high premiums that they could not afford the insurance. Usually individuals living with diabetes, asthma, heart disease, cancer, HIV/AIDS etc. were charged exorbitant amounts for purchase of their own health insurance, thus making it untenable for them to buy and have health insurance coverage. Under the mandates of PPACA, there is a temporary Pre-existing Condition Insurance Plan (PCIP) which would provide health insurance benefits for individuals with preexisting condition who cannot buy or afford private market insurance. The new Pre-existing Condition Insurance Plan under PPACA has currently made it possible for more than 50,000 Americans with preexisting conditions to garner health insurance coverage either through insurance exchanges or their employers. The temporary Pre-existing Condition Insurance Plan helps ensure affordable and available health coverage for individuals who are uninsured because of their preexisting condition. This temporary measure is necessary till 2014 when the effective portion of PPACA mandate that makes it illegal for health insurance companies to discriminate against anyone with a preexisting condition, will take effect.[15] The different states could choose to have their PCIP programs administered either by themselves or by the federal government. The federal program started accepting application for enrollment July 1 2010, while the various states had varied dates for commencement of their enrollment. Thus far 23 states and the District of Columbia have chosen to have their PCIP program administered by the federal government, while 27 states opted to run their own programs.[16]

According to HealthCare.gov, the below chart, indicates the onset of provision of benefits for each state as well as the number of people enrolled within the program as of April 30, 2012.

Table 5.2- Number of People with Coverage by State

State	Federally/State Administered	Date Coverage for Enrollees Began (in 2010)	Number of People Enrolled and with Coverage in Effect Through April 30, 2012
Alabama	Federal	01-Aug	466
Alaska	State	01-Sep	45
Arizona	Federal	01-Aug	2748
Arkansas	State	01-Sep	574

California	State	25-Oct	8662
Colorado	State	01-Sep	1227
Connecticut	State	01-Sep	322
Delaware	Federal	01-Aug	217
District of Columbia	Federal	01-Oct	49
Florida	Federal	01-Aug	5918
Georgia	Federal	01-Aug	2066
Hawaii	Federal	01-Aug	107
Idaho	Federal	01-Aug	590
Illinois	State	01-Sep	2384
Indiana	Federal	01-Aug	1092
Iowa	State	01-Sep	290
Kansas	State	01-Aug	394
Kentucky	Federal	01-Aug	727
Louisiana	Federal	01-Aug	795
Maine	State	01-Aug	41
Maryland	State	01-Sep	959
Massachusetts*	Federal	01-Aug	17
Michigan	State	01-Oct	1263
Minnesota	Federal	01-Aug	424
Mississippi	Federal	01-Aug	260
Missouri	State	15-Aug	1367
Montana	State	01-Aug	317
Nebraska	Federal	01-Aug	266
Nevada	Federal	01-Aug	827
New Hampshire	State	01-Jul	447
New Jersey	State	15-Aug	946
New Mexico	State	01-Aug	1059
New York	State	01-Oct	3320
North Carolina	State	01-Aug	3907
North Dakota	Federal	01-Aug	61
Ohio	State	01-Sep	2598
Oklahoma	State	01-Sep	731
Oregon	State	01-Aug	1344
Pennsylvania	State	01-Oct	5355
Rhode Island	State	15-Sep	166
South Carolina	Federal	01-Aug	1291
South Dakota	State	15-Jul	176
Tennessee	Federal	01-Aug	1191
Texas	Federal	01-Aug	5684
Utah	State	01-Sep	839
Vermont*	Federal	01-Sep	2
Virginia	Federal	01-Aug	1498

Washington	State	01-Sep	782
West Virginia	Federal	01-Sep	113
Wisconsin	State	01-Aug	1373
Wyoming	Federal	01-Aug	185
Total			67,482

Source: HealthCare.Gov. April 2012. [17]

* The two states with asterisks i.e. Massachusetts and Vermont are guarantee issue states, and as such have implemented a significant number of the wider market reforms that are part of the Affordable Care Act that will take effect in 2014. Therefore the two states already offer guaranteed coverage with their commercial health insurance plans that have premiums comparable to PCIP. [18]

Insurance Exchanges

Another inherent part of the health reform Act, is the idea of utilizing affordable Insurance Exchanges, which can be considered one-stop marketplaces, that allows individuals to choose the private health insurance plan that would fit their health insurance needs.[19] The reform requires that by 2014, all the states of the union would have established health insurance exchanges that would select health plans that are qualified to offer coverage. They would also help small employers and individuals obtain coverage. The health plans that would be participating within the exchanges would have one single enrollment form, and the plans would be accredited for quality. They would likewise have to present their benefit options in a standard easy comparison format such that individuals and small businesses can compare health plans and prices. Insurance exchanges would also make it possible for small businesses and individuals to get assistance with regards to questions about insurance plans. The exchanges would also help individuals find out if they are eligible for private insurance tax credits or eligible for health programs like the Children's Health Insurance Program (CHIP). The exchanges are structured to start offering to the public starting from 2014, the same kinds of insurance choices members of Congress will have.[20]

Since the enactment of the federal health care reform law, states across the country have been working to implement the health care mandates, and they can apply for exchange grants up until 2014, to help them pay for the implementation process. Thus so far, as of May 16 2012, $856 million Exchange Establishment Grants have been awarded to 34 states and the District of Columbia to aid in building their exchanges.[21] These grants can be utilized beyond 2014 to provide states with support and time, as they work to build their exchange functionality so as to provide the best exchanges for their residents.

The Grants take into consideration the fact that the different states are making different levels of progress towards establishing exchanges. Thus the grants are structured such that different states can choose based on their needs and planned expenditures when to apply for grant funding. Therefore based on their progress levels, states may initially apply for either level one or level two establishment grants. States that are already ahead in their process of establishing exchanges can apply for level two multi-year establishment grants, while states that are utilizing a more paced step by step approach can apply for level one establishment grants. The level one establishment grant funds for each project year. A thorough examination of state funding request and an analysis of reasonable funding amount from the federal government are crucial prior to award of each state's grant.[22]

According to Healthcare.gov as of May 16, 2012,

- "Forty-nine States and the District of Columbia received up to $1 million in Exchange Planning Grants. Four territories received similar grants on March 21, 2011. States receiving these funds have used them to conduct studies on the feasibility of Exchanges, and conduct community forums to hear directly from residents on how Exchanges should be established.
- Six states and a multi-state consortium led by the University of Massachusetts Medical School received over $241 million in Early Innovator grants to develop model Exchange IT systems. Early Innovator states have committed to assuring that the technology they develop is reusable and transferable to other States. Using the grants, they will develop the building blocks for Exchange IT systems, providing models for how Exchange IT systems can be created."[23]

Below are the different states within the union that have been granted Health Insurance Exchange grants by the federal Government, as of May 16, 2012.

- **Planning Grant Only**
  - Florida (FL)
  - Georgia (GA)
  - Kansas (KS)
  - Louisiana (LA)
  - Montana (MT)
  - New Hampshire (NH)
  - North Dakota (ND)
  - Ohio (OH)
  - Oklahoma (OK)
  - South Carolina (SC)
  - Texas (TX)
  - Utah (UT)
  - Virginia (VA)

- o   Wisconsin (WI)
- o   Wyoming (WY)

- **Planning and Level 1**
  - o   Alabama (AL)
  - o   Arizona (AZ)
  - o   Arkansas (AR)
  - o   California (CA)
  - o   Colorado (CO)
  - o   Connecticut (CT)
  - o   Delaware (DE)
  - o   District of Columbia (DC)
  - o   Hawaii (HI)
  - o   Idaho (ID)
  - o   Illinois (IL)
  - o   Indiana (IN)
  - o   Iowa (IA)
  - o   Kentucky (KY)
  - o   Maine (ME)
  - o   Maryland (MD)
  - o   Massachusetts (MA)
  - o   Michigan (MI)
  - o   Minnesota (MN)
  - o   Mississippi (MS)
  - o   Missouri (MO)
  - o   Nebraska (NE)
  - o   Nevada (NV)
  - o   New Jersey (NJ)
  - o   New Mexico (NM)
  - o   New York (NY)
  - o   North Carolina (NC)
  - o   Oregon (OR)
  - o   Pennsylvania (PA)
  - o   South Dakota (SD)
  - o   Tennessee (TN)
  - o   Vermont (VT)
  - o   West Virginia (WV)

- **Planning, Level 1, Level 2**
  - o   Rhode Island (RI)
  - o   Washington (WA)

- **Territory Establishment Grant**
  - o   American Samoa (AS)

- o Guam (GU)
- o Puerto Rico (PR)
- o Virgin Islands (VI)

- **Did Not Apply**
  - o Alaska (AK)
  - o Federated States of Micronesia (FM)
  - o Marshall Islands (MH)
  - o Northern Mariana Islands (MP)
  - o Palau (PW

Source: HealthCare.Gov May 16, 2012.[24]

Improving and Strengthening Medicare:
PPACA is intended to help enhance Medicare benefits. Medicare is the government health insurance for individuals 65 years or older, for people with end stage renal disease[25] and for individuals with certain disabilities, who are under 65 years old. There are different parts of Medicare that help cover different specific services.

Medicare Part A or Hospital Insurance:
This helps provide coverage for qualified individuals for inpatient hospice, skilled nursing facilities, and home health care and hospitals services. Usually most people do not have to pay a premium for Medicare Part A because the individual or their spouse paid Medicare taxes while they were working within United States. The taxes are usually automatically deducted from paychecks. One can still enroll in Medicare, if they do not automatically get the premium free Part A, but they would have to pay the premiums.[26]

Medicare Part B or Medical Insurance:
Medicare Part B helps provide coverage for some preventive services. It also covers outpatient care, durable medical equipment, home health care, physicians and other health provider services. Eligible individual pay up to the standard monthly Medicare premium, one can buy a private Medicare Supplemental insurance policy (Medigap) so as to have insurance that covers what the original Medicare insurance won't cover.[27]

Medicare Part C Medicare Advantage:
These are Medicare approved private insurance health plan options that allow beneficiaries to get the benefits and services covered under Medicare Part A and B. Some of these plans might also include some extra benefits for extra costs. Medicare Prescription drug coverage (Part d) is usually covered by most Medicare Advantage plans.[28]

Medicare Part D Prescription Drug Coverage:
This covers the cost of most prescription drugs and might actually help lower prescription drug costs. These are run by Medicare approved private insurance companies. Plans vary and so do benefits and costs.[29] There are two main ways of getting Medicare coverage. It is important to note that in addition to the two ways of obtaining Medicare coverage mentioned in the chart on page 91, an eligible individual may also join other types of Medicare plans that are essentially private plans that contracted with Medicare to provide Part A and Part B coverage for Medicare eligible individuals that decide to enroll in such private plans. Such plans include Medicare Advantage plans, Medicare Cost plans, Programs of All-inclusive Care for the Elderly (PACE) and Demonstration/Pilot programs.[30]

There are two main choices for how you get your Medicare coverage. They are shown in a step- by – step diagram below. The two steps demarcate the process of choosing the Medicare plan that is best for the individual.

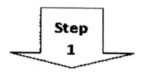

Decide If You Want Original Medicare or a Medicare Advantage Plan

Original Medicare
Part A (Hospital Insurance) and
Part B (Medical Insurance)

- Medicare provides this coverage.
- You have your choice of doctors, hospitals, and other providers that accept Medicare.
- Generally, you or your supplemental coverage pays deductibles and coinsurance.
- You usually pay a monthly premium for Part B.

**Medicare Advantage Plan
(like and HMO or PPO)**
Part C – Includes BOTH Part A (Hospital Insurance) and Part B (Medical Insurance

- Private insurance companies approved by Medicare provide this coverage.
- In most plans, you need to use plan doctors, hospitals, and other providers or you pay more or all of the costs.
- You usually pay a monthly premium (in addition to your Part B premium) and a co-payment or coinsurance for covered services.
- Costs, extra coverage, and rules vary by plan.

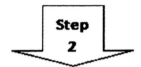

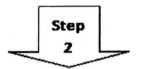

Decide If You Want Prescription Drug Coverage (Part D)

- If you want this coverage, you must choose and join a Medicare Prescription Drug Plan. You usually pay a monthly premium.
- These plans are run by private companies approved by Medicare

Decide If You Want Prescription Drug Coverage (Part D)

- If you want prescription drug coverage, and it's offered by your plan, in most cases you must get it through your plan.
- In some types of plans that don't offer drug coverage, you can join a Medicare Prescription Drug Plan.

Note: If you join a Medicare Advantage Plan, you can't use Medicare Supplement Insurance (Medigap) to pay for out-of-pocket costs you have in a Medicare Advantage Plan. If you already have a Medicare Advantage Plan, you can't be sold a Medigap policy.

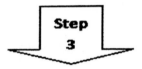

Decide If You Want Supplemental Coverage

- You may want to get coverage that fills gaps in Original Medicare coverage. You can choose to buy a Medicare Supplement Insurance (Medigap) policy from a private company.
- Costs vary by policy and company.
- Employers/unions may offer similar coverage.

Source: Your Medicare Coverage Choices [31]

There are about 50 million older Americans and Americans with disabilities that utilize Medicare on an annual basis. The new health care law is geared towards helping to improve and strengthen Medicare by adding new benefits, fighting fraud, and improving care for patients. The Medicare trust fund is anticipated to be extended to at least 2024 as a result of the expected reduction in waste, fraud, abuse as well as from slowing cost growth in Medicare.[32] The Patient Protection and Affordable Care Act is expected to save the average Medicare beneficiary $4200 over the next ten years and the beneficiaries whose drug costs have hit the "donut hole"[33] will save an average of about $16,000 during the same period. [34] Prior to implementation of PPACA, basic Medicare Part D coverage worked as follows:

> "The beneficiary pays annual Part D monthly Premiums out of pocket and 100% of prescription drug costs until the $310 deductible amount is reached. Once the deductible is reached, beneficiary pays 25% of cost of drugs, while Medicare Part D pays the balance of 75% of the drug costs. After the deductible has been reached, and the total 100% of prescription costs has hit $2,800. That means that the beneficiary has reached their coverage limit, and thus is now responsible for out of pocket cost of future drugs until the beneficiary has reached the yearly out of pocket spending limit of $4,550. Once this limit I reached, the beneficiary is subsequently only responsible for a small amount of the cost of subsequent drugs, usually about 5% of the cost of drugs. The coverage gap between the prescription limit and yearly out of pocket spending limit is referred to as the "donut hole." [35]

The donut hole can represent quite a significant amount of expense for the elderly and the other individuals on Medicare. This is because the individuals within the donut hole usually are the ones with the highest cost of prescription drugs. In some cases it is a choice for them, between paying their mortgage, groceries or buying their prescription medications with their limited income. In some instances as much as 25% of seniors would opt to go without their prescription every year, simply because they could not afford it.[36] But implementation of the Health Care Reform Act, instituted some significant changes that that will help relieve the burden for Medicare beneficiaries that hit the donut hole each year and do not have Medicare Extra Help.[37]

Lower Cost Prescription Drugs:
Starting from June 2010, when a Medicare beneficiary enters the Part D donut hole, the individual will receive a onetime $250 rebate check. Nearly four million Medicare beneficiaries within the donut hole received the $250 check in 2010, to help them with their prescription costs. Then from 2011, beneficiaries in the donut hole, will receive 50% discount on brand name drugs and will pay less for generic Part D drugs. A total of $2.1 billion worth of 50% brand name prescription discount was received by 3.6 Medicare beneficiaries within the donut hole, in 2011. That is an average savings of $604 per person discount. From 2013, beneficiaries in the donut hole, will gradually pay less for brand-name Part D prescription drugs, and by 2020, there would be no more coverage gap or donut hole. Subsequently beneficiaries will only pay 25% of the costs of prescription drugs until they reach the yearly out of pocket spending limit.

Throughout this period, the beneficiary will continue to receive Medicare Part D coverage for prescription drugs so long as the individual is on a prescription drug plan.[38] This will go a long way towards helping Medicare beneficiaries save money and at the same time get the prescription medications that they need to manage their health.

Free Preventive Services:
One of the requirements of the new health care law, is that recommended preventive health care services for Medicare recipients i.e. diabetes, high blood pressure screenings, flu shots, Tobacco cessation counseling[39] and a new Annual Wellness Visit for seniors will now be covered free of charge. Established Medicare beneficiaries, under the health plan, will receive a yearly wellness visit to update or develop a personalized prevention plan that is based on the individual's current health and risk factors. For newly enrolled Medicare beneficiaries, they will be eligible for a free with no cost sharing one time annual review of their health, this review would also involve education and counseling about preventive services and other care.[40] Thus far about 32.5 million seniors have already received one or more preventive services. For the covered screenings there will be no more Medicare Part B deductible or copayment, if they meet certain coverage criteria. There is no pay for preventive services if the individual is an established Medicare patient, but for newly enrolled Medicare beneficiaries, they will have to wait 12 month after their initial welcome enrollment preventive visit. Also, some beneficiaries might have to pay co-insurance for the office visit incident to the preventive checkup. Some enrollees within Medicare Advantage Plan might not have the benefits free.

The following preventive services are available under the new reform law.

Abdominal Aortic Aneurysm Screenings:
This is a one-time screening ultrasound for people at risk.

Alcohol Misuse Counseling:
Medicare covers one alcohol misuse screening per year. Counseling may be covered if your screening result is positive.

Bone Mass Measurements:
This measurement checks the risk for broken bones. This service is covered once every 24 months (more often if medically necessary) for people who have certain medical conditions or meet certain criteria.

Cardiovascular Disease (Behavioral Therapy):
Medicare covers one visit per year to help lower risk for cardiovascular disease. During this visit, the physician may discuss aspirin use (if appropriate), check

the patient's blood pressure, and provide healthy eating tips for the Medicare enrollee or patient.

Cardiovascular Screenings:
This particular screening helps detect conditions that may lead to a heart attack or stroke. This service is covered every five years and it involves testing the patient's cholesterol, lipid, and triglyceride levels.

Colon Cancer Screenings (Colorectal):
Medicare covers colorectal screening tests to help find pre-cancerous polyps (growths in the colon) so they can be removed before they turn into cancer.

Depression Screenings:
Medicare covers depression screenings by the Medicare patient's primary care doctor once every 12 months.

Diabetes Screenings:
Diabetes screenings are covered if you have any of the following risk factors: high blood pressure (hypertension), history of abnormal cholesterol and triglyceride levels (dyslipidemia), obesity, or a history of high blood sugar (glucose). Based on the results of these tests, the individual may be eligible for up to two diabetes screenings every year.

Diabetes Self-Management Training:
For individuals that have diabetes, the patient's doctor or other health care provider must provide a written order, regarding how to manage the diabetes so as to reduce possible complications. The order would be explained clearly to the patient, with the goal of teaching the patient how to control their diabetes and as such, the order would help the patient follow the guidelines to help manage the diabetic condition.

EKG Screenings:
Medicare covers a one-time screening EKG if the individual gets a referral for it as a result of the one-time "Welcome to Medicare" Preventive Visit.

Flu Shots:
Flu shots are covered once a flu season, either in the fall or winter for Medicare beneficiaries.

Glaucoma Tests:
This type of eye test is covered once every 12 months for any Medicare enrollee that is at high risk for glaucoma.

Hepatitis B Shots:
This is covered for people at high or medium risk for Hepatitis B. The risk for Hepatitis B increases if an individual has hemophilia, End-Stage Renal Disease (ESRD), or a condition that increases the risk for infection. Other factors may increase the risk for Hepatitis B, so learning about the other factors that contribute to risk of hepatitis will help Medicare enrollees possibly mitigate their risks. Enrollees pay 20% of the Medicare-approved amount, and the Part B deductible applies.

HIV Screenings:
Medicare covers HIV screening for people with Medicare who are pregnant and people at increased risk for the infection. Medicare also covers the screening for anyone who asks for the test.

Mammograms:
Mammograms are covered by Medicare, once every 12 months for all women enrolled in Medicare aged 40 years and older. Medicare covers one baseline mammogram for women between ages 35–39.

Medical Nutrition Therapy Services:
Medicare may also cover medical nutrition therapy and certain related services if the individual has diabetes or kidney disease, or if the person has had a kidney transplant within in the last 36 months, and their doctor had referred the person for the service.

Obesity Screening and Counseling:
If a Medicare beneficiary, has a body mass index of 30 or more, Medicare would cover intensive counseling to help the individual lose weight. This counseling may be covered if it is received within a primary care setting, where it can be coordinated with a comprehensive prevention plan.

Pap Tests and Pelvic Exams:
Medicare covers Pap smears and Pelvic exams once every 24 months for women with normal past Pap tests and exams or once every 12 months for women at high risk, as well as for women of child-bearing age who have had an exam that indicated cancer or other abnormalities within the past 3 years.

Preventive Visits:
Medicare covers two types of preventive visits, an initial preventive visit for new Medicare enrollees and a preventive visit each subsequent year after that.

Pneumococcal Shots:
Medicare also covers pneumococcal shots for beneficiaries, though most people only need this preventive shot once in their lifetime.

Prostate Cancer Screenings:
Medicare covers a digital rectal exam and Prostate Specific Antigen (PSA) test
once every 12 months for all men with Medicare over age 50.

Sexually Transmitted Infections Screening and Counseling:
Medicare covers sexually transmitted infection (STI) screenings for chlamydia,
gonorrhea, syphilis, and/or Hepatitis B for people who meet certain criteria.
Medicare also covers up to two individuals 20 to 30 minutes, face-to-face, high-
intensity behavioral counseling sessions each year for people who meet certain
criteria.

Smoking Cessation (counseling to stop smoking):
Medicare covers smoking cessation counseling as a preventive service and the
enrollee will not pay any fess for the counseling sessions. Source: Medi-
care.Gov, Preventive Services.[41]

Part of the provisions of the new health care law utilizes tougher screening procedures, stronger penalties as well as new technology in the fight against health
care fraud. As such the federal government has partnered with state and private
organizations with the goals of stopping fraudulent health care practices, with
the eventual goal of performing sophisticated analytics on a healthcare industry-
wide data set that will detect and predict fraud schemes. The partnership is a
voluntary one formed out of the need to prevent frauds and safeguard health care
dollars so as to save health care consumers and taxpayers' money. There is also
an attendant goal of revealing and stopping scams that cut across a number of
public and private payers.[42] As a direct result of some of these efforts, $10.7
billion was recovered over the last 3 years and in 2011 alone, $4.1 billion in
taxpayer dollars were recovered.

There have also been an increased number of individuals charged with
fraud, from 821 in 2008 to 1,430 in 2011. That is an almost 75% increase.[43] It is
important to have these screening procedures in place, because both Medicare
and Medicaid health care fraud has cost billions of dollars in health care costs.
These medical fraud scams run the gamut from billing for healthcare services
that were not provided, to fraudulent billings for durable medical equipment.
The Medicare Fraud Strike Force that was established by the federal government
in 2007, randomly visited about 1600 health care offices in Miami and found
that nearly a third of the businesses, about 481, were not in existence, yet they
had billed Medicare $237 million dollars the previous year for durable medical
equipment.[44] Likewise federal authorities announced in May, 2012 that they had
arrested 107 healthcare providers, including doctors and nurses over several
cities and charged them with defrauding Medicare of $452 million.[45] Medicare
fraud is so lucrative that even members of the Russian and Nigerian mobs[46] as
well as New York mafias are involved in scams involving defrauding Medicare.[47] Thus better fraud screening measures proffer the opportunity to cut down
massive amounts of fiscal waste due to fraudulent Medicare billings and scams.

Improving Care Coordination and Quality:
This is to be carried out by the recently established Center for Medicare and Medicaid Innovation which was established by the implementation of the Affordable Care Plan. The Center was established with the goals of identifying, developing, supporting and evaluating advanced new and efficient methods of health care delivery and payment for Medicare, Medicaid, and Children's Health Insurance Program (CHIP). This process will be affected in an open, transparent and competitive manner with the end focus of improving the health care system for all Americans.[48] The Mission of the Center for Medicare and Medicaid Innovation reads as follows:

- "Better health care by improving all aspects of patient care, including Safety, Effectiveness, Patient-Centeredness, Timeliness, Efficiency, and Equity (the domains of quality in patient care as defined by the Institute of Medicine).
- Better health by encouraging healthier lifestyles in the entire population, including increased physical activity, better nutrition, avoidance of behavioral risks, and wider use of preventative care.
- Lower costs through improvement by promoting preventative medicine, improved coordination of health care services, and by reducing waste and inefficiencies. These efforts will reduce the national cost of health care and lower out-of-pocket expenses for all Medicare, Medicaid, and CHIP beneficiaries."[49]

As can be seen from their mission statement there is an expanded focus on prevention as well as efficiency in Health service delivery.

Providing Choices for Medicaid Recipients while lowering costs:
Since the implementation of the Affordable Care Act, in 2010 through 2012, Medicare Advantage plan has seen its enrollment increase by 17 percent, while subsequently providing more choice for seniors and decreasing premiums for the plans by 16 percent. Such gains call into question the financing of the health care reform plan. Since the goal of the health reform plan is to expand coverage for everyone, including both the uninsured and the uninsurable, plus the provision of more services, the question that begs to be asked is how that is going to be achieved without massive increased costs.

Financing of the Affordable Care Act

The Patient Protection and Affordable Care Act was enacted with the broad goals of expanding care while at the same time reducing costs associated with uninsured care. Some of the political portrayals of the reform Act focus on the notion, that it would greatly add to the national deficit and the costs associated therein with implementation and expansion of coverage would add to the federal deficit and thus be untenable for the government to maintain. But according to Richard S. Foster, Office of the Actuary, Center for Medicare and Medicaid Services, the health insurance reform would not be a fiscal disaster as some predict. The chart on the next page is a report detailing expected costs of implementation of the reform plan. The chart should be read with the understanding that most of the provisions of the reform act, take effect 6 years out of the 10 year budget period.

Figure 5.1- Estimated Effects of the Patient Protection and Affordable Care Act, as Enacted and Amended on Enrollment by Insurance Coverage (In Millions)

Provisions	2010	2011	2012	2013	2014	2015	2016	2017	2018	2019	Total, FY 2010-2019
Total*	\$9.2	-\$0.7	-\$12.6	-\$22.3	\$16.8	\$57.9	\$63.1	\$54.2	\$47.2	\$38.5	\$251.3
Coverage Provisions:											
Medicaid Expansion and CHIP Funding	3.3	4.6	4.9	5.2	82.9	119.2	138.2	146.6	157.6	165.8	832.2
Credits:	—	—	—	—	38.8	62.9	78.7	72.2	76.3	81.2	410.3
Individual Exchange Subsidies:	3.3	4.6	4.9	5.2	49.6	67.6	77.9	99.1	110.3	115.5	537.9
Refundable Premium Tax Credits	—	—	—	—	43.9	61.4	76.3	99.1	110.3	115.5	506.5
Reduced Cost Sharing Requirements	—	—	—	—	38.4	54.2	68.3	88.6	98.7	103.0	451.1
Small Employer Credits	3.3	4.6	4.9	5.2	3.5	7.2	8.0	10.5	11.6	12.5	55.4
Penalties:	—	—	—	—	5.7	6.2	1.6	0.0	0.0	0.0	31.4
Individual Penalties	—	—	—	—	-5.5	-11.3	-18.4	-24.7	-29.0	-30.9	-119.9
Employer Penalties	—	—	—	—	0.0	-2.4	-3.3	-7.6	-4.6	-9.2	-33.1
	—	—	—	—	-5.5	-9.0	-13.0	-17.1	-20.4	-21.8	-56.8
Medicare	-1.2	-4.7	-14.9	-26.3	-43.8	-60.3	-75.2	-92.1	-108.2	-125.7	-575.1
Medicaid/CHIP (Excluding Coverage Expansions)	-0.9	-0.9	0.3	4.5	8.6	5.1	4.6	3.4	1.3	1.7	28.3
Cost Trend Proposals:											
Comparative Effectiveness Research	—	—	—	—	0.0	-0.1	-0.2	-0.4	-0.6	-0.9	-3.3
Prevention and Wellness	—	—	—	—	0.0	-0.1	-0.2	-0.4	-0.6	-0.9	-3.3
Fraud and Abuse	—	—	—	—	0.0	0.0	0.0	0.0	0.0	0.0	0.0
Administrative Simplification	—	—	—	—	0.0	0.0	0.0	0.0	0.0	0.0	0.0
Additional Proposals:	5.6	0.4	-3.3	-5.6	-5.9	-6.0	-4.3	-3.4	-2.8	-3.4	-27.8
CLASS Program	—	-2.8	-4.5	-5.6	-5.9	-6.0	-4.3	-3.4	-2.8	-2.4	-37.8
Immediate Reforms	5.6	2.2	1.2	—	—	—	—	—	—	—	10.0

* Excludes Title IX revenue provisions except for sections 9008 (fees on manufacturers and importers of brand-name prescription drugs) and 9015 (additional HI payroll tax). Also excludes certain provisions with limited impacts and Federal administrative costs.

† Excludes the Medicare impact of CER, which is included in the Medicare savings total.

Source: Richard S. Foster, Office of the Actuary, Center for Medicare and Medicaid Services, Department of Health and Human Service.[50]

Figure 5.2- Estimated Cost of the Reform through 2019[51]

Prior Law Baseline	Calendar Year									
	2010	2011	2012	2013	2014	2015	2016	2017	2018	2019
Medicare	46.9	48.0	49.4	50.9	52.4	53.9	55.4	57.1	58.7	60.5
Medicaid CHIP	59.2	60.5	61.6	62.0	60.6	60.3	61.1	61.9	62.7	63.5
Other Public	12.3	12.6	12.9	13.2	13.6	13.9	14.2	14.6	14.9	15.2
Employer-Sponsored Private Health Insurance	163.8	163.2	164.5	165.0	166.1	166.6	166.4	166.2	166.0	165.9
Other Private Health Insurance*	26.1	25.3	25.5	25.6	25.8	25.8	25.8	25.8	25.8	25.7
Uninsured	48.3	48.6	47.9	48.1	50.0	51.7	53.1	54.4	55.6	56.9
Insured Share of US Population†	84.4%	84.5%	84.8%	84.9%	84.4%	84.0%	83.8%	83.5%	83.3%	83.0%

New Law — PPACA	Calendar Year									
	2010	2011	2012	2013	2014	2015	2016	2017	2018	2019
Medicare	46.9	48.0	49.4	50.9	52.4	53.9	55.4	57.1	58.7	60.5
Medicaid CHIP	59.2	60.5	61.6	62.0	83.6	84.6	84.1	82.1	82.9	83.9
Other Public	12.6	12.6	12.9	13.2	13.6	13.9	14.2	14.6	14.9	15.2
Employer-sponsored Private Health Insurance	164.3	163.7	164.9	165.5	168.1	169.0	166.6	164.7	163.7	164.5
Other Private Health Insurance*	26.1	25.3	25.5	25.6	12.6	12.2	11.5	10.9	10.4	10.0
Exchanges	—	—	—	—	16.9	18.6	24.8	29.8	31.4	31.6
Uninsured	47.5	48.1	47.4	47.6	23.8	22.2	21.0	22.0	22.8	23.1
Insured Share of US Population†	84.7%	84.6%	85.0%	85.0%	92.6%	93.2%	93.6%	93.3%	93.1%	93.1%

Impact of PPACA	Calendar Year									
	2010	2011	2012	2013	2014	2015	2016	2017	2018	2019
Medicare	—	—	—	—	—	—	—	—	—	—
Medicaid CHIP	—	—	—	—	23.0	24.3	23.1	20.2	20.2	20.4
Other Public	0.4	—	—	—	—	—	—	—	—	—
Employer-sponsored Private Health Insurance	0.5	0.5	0.5	0.5	2.0	2.5	0.2	-1.5	-2.4	-1.4
Other Private Health Insurance*	—	—	—	—	-13.2	-13.7	-14.3	-14.9	-15.3	-15.7
Exchanges	—	—	—	—	16.9	18.6	24.8	29.8	31.4	31.6
Uninsured	-0.9	-0.5	-0.5	-0.5	-26.2	-29.5	-32.1	-32.4	-32.9	-33.8
Insured Share of US Population†	0.3%	0.2%	0.2%	0.2%	8.2%	9.1%	9.8%	9.8%	9.9%	10.1%

* In the prior-law baseline, other private health insurance includes private Medicare supplemental coverage and individual coverage. In the new-law estimates, other private health insurance includes only those with Medicare supplemental coverage

† Calculated as a proportion of total U.S. population, including unauthorized immigrants.

Figure 5.3- Estimated Effects of the Patient Protection and Affordable Care Act, as Enacted and Amended on Enrollment by Insurance Coverage (in billions)

Provisions	Fiscal Year										Total, 2010-19
	2010	2011	2012	2013	2014	2015	2016	2017	2018	2019	
Total*	$9.2	–$0.7	–$12.6	–$22.3	$16.8	$57.9	$63.1	$54.2	$47.2	$38.5	$251.3
Coverage†	3.3	4.6	4.9	5.2	82.9	119.2	138.2	146.6	157.6	165.8	828.2
Medicare	1.2	–4.7	–14.9	–26.3	–68.8	–60.3	–75.2	–92.1	–108.2	–125.7	–575.1
Medicaid/CHIP	–0.9	–0.9	0.8	4.5	8.6	5.1	4.6	3.4	1.3	1.7	28.3
Cost trend‡	—	—	—	—	–0.0	–0.1	–0.2	–0.4	–0.6	–0.9	–2.3
CLASS program	—	–2.8	–4.5	–5.6	–5.9	–6.0	–4.3	–3.4	–2.8	–2.4	–37.8
Immediate reforms	5.6	3.2	1.2	—	—	—	—	—	—	—	10.0

* Excludes Title IX revenue provisions except for sections 9008 and 9015, certain provisions with limited impacts, and Federal administrative costs.

† Includes expansion of Medicaid eligibility and additional funding for CHIP.

‡ Includes estimated non-Medicare Federal savings from provisions for comparative effectiveness research, prevention and wellness, fraud and abuse, and administrative simplification. Excludes impacts of other provisions that would affect cost growth rates, such as the productivity adjustments to Medicare payment rates (which are reflected in the Medicare line) and the section 9001 excise tax on high-cost employer plans.

The above chart[52] shows that the total estimated costs of the reform with the included Medicaid expansion and increased Chip funding through fiscal year 2019 to be $828.2 billion. The immediate reform provisions are expected to result in net savings of about $577 billion therefore resulting in a net cost of $251 billion during this fiscal period. But the reform program is also expected to have some sources of revenue from excise tax on high cost employer provided health insurance coverage as well as from other revenue provisions of the reform plan.[53] Accordingly the Joint Committee on Taxation (JCT) and the Congressional Budget Office (CBO) have estimated that the cost of the health reform provisions would be more than offset by net amount of Medicare savings as well as the additional tax and other revenues, thereby resulting in a reduction of the federal deficit through 2019.[54] The general contention is that the upholding of the health reform Act will result in a net federal saving and as such help reduce the federal deficit. Figure 5.5 on the next page showcases that contention:

Figure 5.4

**Major Effects on the Federal Budget in 2022 of Changes in
Medicaid Enrollment Due to the Recent Supreme Court Decision**

(Billions of dollars)

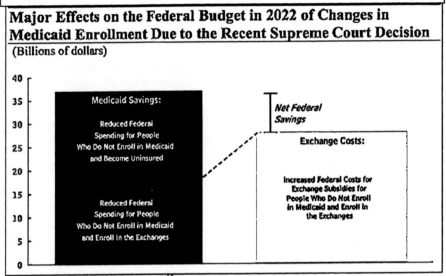

Source: Forbes July 24, 2012. [55]

Likewise the CBO and JCT now estimate that over the 2012-2021 period there would be a projected decrease of about $50 billion from the original March 2011 estimated PPACA cost of implementation. The new net cost of PPACA implementation is now about $1.083 trillion for the 10 year period. [56] The costs include Medicaid, Children's Health Insurance program (CHIP), tax credits costs and other subsidies for health insurance purchases through the recently established insurance exchanges, subsequent costs as well as tax credits for small employers. These costs are estimated to add up to about $1.5 trillion. [57] On the other hand there would be revenue receipts of about $0.4 trillion, which would offset some of the $1.5 trillion, estimated implementation costs of PPACA. The revenue receipts are projected to be derived as mentioned earlier from the new excise tax on high premium insurance plans, penalty payments as well as increases in tax revenue. It is important to note that these estimated budgetary figures does not factor in federal administrative costs, nor does it factor in provisions of the law that would generate added tax revenue as well as greatly reduce Medicare spending from what it was prior to the implementation of the law.[58]

Some of the changes with regards to the projected expenses of the reform plan implementation were due to new legislation, changes in economic outlook and technical changes. There were several laws that were enacted in 2011 that changed the projected budgetary outlook. Some of the new laws had an impact on the projection of the expenditures for the health reform law. There were three main legislations by lawmakers that had an impact on the budgetary outlook for implementation of the health care act. The three pieces of legislation modified coverage provisions of the Affordable Care Act. According to the Congressional Budget Office, There was;

"1) The Three Percent Withholding Repeal and Job Creation Act (P.L. 112-56) adds nontaxable Social Security benefits to the definition of modified adjusted gross income for the purposes of determining eligibility for cer tain applicants for Medicaid and for subsidies for health insurance pur chased through the exchanges. That change reduced the number of indi viduals who will qualify for Medicaid and increased the number who will qualify for subsidies through the exchanges. CBO and JCT estimated that the legislation will reduce the costs of the ACA's insurance coverage pro visions by $13 billion over the 2012–2021 period. That estimate includes a reduction of $33 billion in spending for Medicaid and an increase of $15 billion in costs for exchange subsidies over the 2012–2021 period, along with other effects that will increase deficits by an estimated $5 billion. (The budgetary effects of this legislation were incorporated in CBO's Jan uary 2012 baseline).

2) The Comprehensive 1099 Taxpayer Protection and Repayment of Ex change Subsidy Overpayments Act of 2011 (P.L. 112-9) includes a provi sion that was estimated to reduce the costs of the ACA's insurance cover age provisions by about $25 billion over the 2012–2021 period, mostly through reductions in the net costs of providing subsidies for purchasing health insurance through the exchanges. (The budgetary effects of this leg islation were incorporated in CBO's August 2011 baseline).

3) The Department of Defense and Full-Year Continuing Appropriations Act of 2011 (P.L. 112-10) repealed the Free Choice Voucher program, which provided a mechanism through which certain employees could use their employer's health insurance contribution to purchase coverage through the exchanges. CBO and JCT estimated that repealing this provision will in crease revenues by $0.4 billion over the 2012–2021 period. (The budget ary effects of this legislation were also incorporated in CBO's August 2011 baseline)." [59]

Thus the above mentioned legislations, by their very nature increased the possi ble revenues that would be garnered through the Affordable Care Act. These legislations changed some of the budgetary estimates of CBO and JCT. Like wise there have been changes made to the 2011 Economic outlooks for USA, the 2012 CBO's economic outlook forecast delineates a slower recovery than the one previously forecast for 2011. This had an impact on the projected costs of PPACA implementation. CBO and JCT based on their estimation of slower eco nomic recovery, made attendant technical changes to their estimating proce dures. [60]

Both the CBO and JCT reports also show that there are more uninsured non-elderly adults than was previously estimated and more people are now ex pected to get their health insurance coverage from Medicaid or Children's

Health Insurance Program (CHIP) than from their employers or insurance exchanges. The expectation is that more individuals are going to be uninsured than previously estimated.[61] The health reform plan is expected to decrease the number of nonelderly uninsured by 30 million to only 33 million uninsured by 2016 and in subsequently years further reduce that number to between 26 to 27 uninsured. This is expected to increase the percentage of nonelderly insured individuals to 82 percent in 2012, and 93 percent in 2016 and subsequent years. Likewise CBO and JCT estimate that from 2016 and thereafter, there would be about 3-5 million people less that would be enrolled within employer provided health insurance than prior to the implementation of the law. Also for 2016 and beyond, implementation of PPACA would result in about 20-23 million people receiving their coverage through health insurance exchanges while about 16-17 million more people would be enrolled within Medicaid and CHIP. [62]

---

1. A More Secure Future: What the New Health Law Means for You and Your Family. (n.d.). Retrieved July 23, 2012, from The White House: http://www.whitehouse.gov/healthreform/healthcare-overview#consumer-rights

2. Children's Pre-existing Conditions. (2012, July 23). Retrieved July 23, 2012, from HealthCare.gov: http://www.healthcare.gov/law/features/rights/childrens-pre-existing-conditions/index.html

3. A grandfathered health insurance plan for the purposes of PPACA, is a Health insurance plan in which an individual was enrolled in by the date of PPACA enactment i.e. on March 23rd 2010. So as long as an individual was enrolled in a health insurance plan as of March 23 2010 , the insurance is grandfathered. Grandfathered health plans are subject only to a few requirements under PPACA with differing effective dates.

4. Fernandez, B. (2010, June 7). Grandfathered Health Plans Under the Patient Protection and Affordable Care Act. Retrieved July 30, 2012, from National Conference of State Legislators: http://www.ncsl.org/documents/health/GrandfatheredPlans.pdf

5. Ibid

6. Ibid

7. A More Secure Future: What the New Health Law Means for you and Your Family

8. Ibid

9. National Conference of State Legislatures

10. A More Secure Future: What the New Health Law Means for you and Your Family.

11. National Conference of State Legislatures

12. Ibid

13. Ibid

14. Ibid

15. A More Secure Future: What the New Health Law Means for you and Your Family.

16. State by State Enrollment in the Preexisting Insurance Plan. (2012, April 30). Retrieved July 26, 2012, from HealthCare.gov: http://www.healthcare.gov/news/ fact-sheets/2012/06/pcip06152012a.html

17. Ibid

18. Ibid

19. A More Secure Future: What the New Health Law Means for you and Your Family.

20. Ibid

21. More States Work to Implement Health Care Law. (2012, May 16). Retrieved July 25, 2012, from U.S. Department of Health and Human Services: http://www.hhs.gov/news/press/2012pres/05/2012/20120516a.html
22. Creating a New Competitive Marketplace: Affordable Insurance Exchanges. (2012, May 16). Retrieved July 25, 2012, from HealthCare.gov: http://www.healthcare.gov/news/factsheets/2011/05/exchanges05232011a.html
23. Ibid
24. Ibid
25. End stage renal disease occurs when a person's kidneys have failed permanently thereby requiring dialysis or kidney transplant.
26. What is Medicare?
27. Ibid
28. Ibid
29. Ibid
30. Your Medicare Coverage Choices. (n.d.). Retrieved June 29, 2012, from Medicare.gov: http://www.medicare.gov/navigation/medicare-basics/coverage-choices.aspx
31. Ibid
32. A More Secure Future: What the New Health Law Means for You and Your Family.
33. The Medicare Donut hole can be defined as the coverage gap that occurs once a beneficiary has spent the maximum limit allowed by Medicare for prescription medicines for that particular beneficiary. Once that limit has been reached, the beneficiary will have to pay the total costs of prescribed medicines out of pocket until the catastrophic limit is reached. For example for 2009 , prior to the enactment of PPACA, if your Medicare prescription coverage limit is $3275 and you have reached that limit, i.e. Medicare has covered that amount for you for your prescription medicines, any further expenditures for prescription medicines would have to be covered out of pocket by you.
34. A More Secure Future: What the New Health Law Means for You and Your Family.
35. Blum, J. (2012, August 9). What is the Donut Hole? Retrieved July 27, 2012, from HealthCare.gov: http://www.healthcare.gov/blog/2010/08/donuthole.html
36. A More Secure Future: What the New Health Law Means for You and Your Family
37. According to Medicare.Gov, Medicare and Social Security can help Medicare beneficiaries with limited income and resources, through a program that helps them pay for their prescription drugs. Qualified beneficiaries could pay only between $1-$6 for each drug. Source: Medicare Prescription Drug Coverage Part D. (n.d.). Retrieved July 27, 2012, from http://www.medicare.gov/navigation/medicare-basics/medicare-benefits/part-d.aspx?AspxAutoDetectCookieSupport=1#CoverageGap
38. Blum
39. The Tobacco Cessation counseling under the health reform law is now free of charge regardless of if you have been diagnosed with an illness caused or complicated by tobacco use. But the coinsurance and deductible will still apply for your treatment of a tobacco related disease if you have been diagnosed as having a tobacco related disease.
40. Medicare Preventive Services. (2012, July 28). Retrieved July 28, 2012, from Healthcare.gov: http://www.healthcare.gov/law/features/65-older/medicare-preventive-services/index.html
41. Ibid
42. New Tools to Fight Fraud, Strengthen Federal and Private Health Programs, and Protect Consumer and Taxpayers Dollars. (2012, July 28). Retrieved July 28, 2012, from Healthcare.gov: http://www.healthcare.gov/news/factsheets/2012/02/medicare-fraud02142012a.html

43. A More Secure Future: What the New Health Law Means for You and Your Family
44. Mathews, M. (2012, May 31). Medicare and Medicaid Fraud Is Costing Taxpayers Billions.   Retrieved   July   28,   2012,   from   Forbes: http://www.forbes.com/sites/merrillmatthews/2012/05/31/medicare-and-medicaid-fraud-is-costing-taxpayers-billions/
45. Ibid
46. Ibid
47. Capo. (2009, October 15). Florida Bonanno Crime Family Members Admit Guilt. Retrieved July 29, 2012, from Mafiatoday.com: http://mafiatoday.com/bonanno-family/florida-bonanno-crime-family-members-admit-guilt/
48 Center for Medicare and Medicaid Services. (2012, July 24). Retrieved July 30, 2012, from CMS.gov: http://innovations.cms.gov/
49. Ibid
50. Foster
51. Ibid
52. Ibid
53. Ibid
54. Ibid
55. Roy, A. (2012, July 24). CBO Guesstimates that the Supreme Court's Impact on ObamaCare   is   Modest.   Retrieved   August   3,   2012,   from   Forbes: http://www.forbes.com/sites/aroy/2012/07/24/cbo-guesstimates-that-ObamaCare-will-cover-3-million-less-people-after-the-supreme-court-saving-84-billion/
56 CBO Releases Updated Estimates for the Insurance Coverage Provisions of the Affordable Care Act. (2012, March 13). Retrieved August 3, 2012, from Congressional Budget Office: http://www.cbo.gov/publication/43080
57 Ibid.
58 Ibid.
59. Updated Estimates for the Insurance Coverage Provisions of the Affordable Care Act. (2012, March). Retrieved January 10, 2013, from Congressional Budget Office: http://www.cbo.gov/sites/default/files/cbofiles/attachments/03-13-Coverage%20Estimates.pdf
60. CBO Releases Updated Estimates for the Insurance Coverage Provisions of the Affordable Care Act
61. Ibid
62. Ibid

Chapter 6

Health Insurance Providers in Tennessee

Health Insurance Provider's Perspectives

So how is the Affordable Care Act going to Impact health insurance companies in Tennessee, and the nation in general? How are health care companies in Tennessee and in the nation dealing with the requirements of the Act? As of August 2012, there are fifteen insurance companies that provide health coverage in Tennessee. The companies are as follows: Aetna life Insurance Company, American Republic Insurance, Blue Cross and Blue Shield of Tennessee, Celtic Insurance, Connecticut General Life Insurance Company (CIGNA), Coventry Health and Life Insurance Company, Freedom Life Insurance Company of America, Golden Rule Insurance, Guarantee Trust Life Insurance, Humana Insurance Company, Independence American Insurance Company, MEGA Life and Health Insurance Company, National Foundation Life Insurance Company , Time Insurance which is the same as Unified Life Insurance company and finally World Insurance Company. The scope of services of Aetna insurance company, which is one of the largest providers of health insurance companies, will be discussed here for an idea of the basis of coverage of insurance companies in Tennessee. This chapter will also discuss how the mandates of the Affordable Care Act would possibly impact health insurance companies within Tennessee and USA in general.

Aetna life insurance Company is a New York Stock Exchange (NYSE) traded insurance company that is based in Connecticut that provide health care, dental, pharmacy, group life, and disability insurance, as well as employee benefits for small, medium and large employers within the 50 states. As of August 2012, the company provides health insurance coverage for all dependent children up to age 26 except in Ohio, where coverage can be provided for dependents up to age 28 and in Florida and Nebraska, where dependent coverage is provided up to age 30. The company does not provide coverage for pre-existing conditions for applicants that are over 19 years old, but this aspect of the health insurance plan would be obsolete when the Patient Protection and Affordable Care Plan goes fully into effect in 2014.

Pre-Existing Conditions

The plan delineates that 19 or older applicants, with pre-existing conditions during the initial 12 months of their effective date of coverage will not have their treatment for such conditions covered, unless they had prior continuous coverage for at least 63 days immediately prior to signing the new insurance application.

Aetna provides health insurance services for Tennessee residents. According to the company's online site, there are 18.029 million medical enrollees, 13.590 million dental enrollees and 8.661 million pharmacy members. The health insurance company likewise has more than 1 million healthcare professionals as part of the caregivers that provide health services to their enrollees. About 582,000 of their health care professionals are primary care doctors and specialists, and they have more than 5,400 hospitals within their plan network. The company also has a network of specialist physicians that are Aexcel[1] recognized, based on their clinical performance and cost efficiency.[2] Aetna enrollees can usually choose without a referral specialists from 12 different health care categories, namely Cardiology, Cardiothoracic surgery, Vascular surgery, Urology, Gastroenterology, General surgery, Neurology, Neurosurgery, Plastic Surgery, Otolaryngology/ENT, Obstetrics & Gynecology and Orthopedics. Enrollees can sometimes actually save costs by choosing these specialists that are Aexcel recognized.[3]

Aetna utilizes an extensive process in determining which doctors are to be Aexcel recognized. It is important to note that Aetna has doctors within their plans that are not Aexcel recognized, although all doctors within their plan are included within the clinical evaluations utilized to designate Aexcel Performance status. In order to be recognized as such, their doctors must have treated a certain number of patients within their specialties as well as have passed clinical performance criteria. There are five performance categories of measure, including claim based measures. An Aetna doctor must have seen at least 10 Aetna cases for each specific applicable measure or no less than 30 Aetna cases for all evaluated measures. The hospital readmission rates after 30 days is also considered for the specialist as well as rates of health care complications during hospital care. Other considerations for clinical performance include whether the specialist utilized other treatments that have been shown to improve outcomes for that particular specialty. Considerations are also given for doctors' utilization of current health care technology, external recognition and participation in activities that are related to maintenance of the doctor's medical board certification.[4]

These standards for Aexcel designation, were derived from guidelines from differing medical National Associations., including, National Quality Forum, American Heart Association, American College of Obstetricians and Gynecologists, Agency for Health Research and Quality, Ambulatory Care Quality Alliance, American Board of Medical Specialties, American Osteopathic Association, The National Committee for Quality Assurance, Center for Medicare & Medicaid Services, and the Society of Thoracic Surgeons Centers. Most doctors usually follow the guidelines, as a routine part of their medical practice , as such there is a seamless integration of the standards required of the doctors, especially considering that doctors within the network have to go through extensive Credentialing prior to joining Aetna. Doctors that do not meet the basic Aexcel designation requirements are not evaluated for the next step, but they can still be part of the Aetna provider network. [5]

In order to evaluate efficiency for the specialists, total costs of services by the specialist are considered. Current specialists within the plan, who have managed at least 20 episodes of care for Aetna enrollees during the past three years, are identified. The cost, number and type of services provided by the specialists are identified, as well as review of inpatient, outpatient, diagnostic, laboratory and pharmacy claims.[6]

Aetna provides different insurance plans, for its members to choose from. The different plans are The High Deductible Preferred Provider Organization (PPO), the Preferred Provider Organization (PPO), Preferred Provider Organization (PPO) Value and the Preventive and Hospital Care.[7] It is important to note that Aetna also offers Aetna HMO but only in Pennsylvania. So Aetna HMO will not be discussed within this book since it is not offered in Tennessee.

The High Deductible Preferred Provider Organization (PPO), can be chosen by individuals that want to pay lower premiums, but in order to pay lower premiums the deductibles are higher. This type of insurance can be coupled with Health Savings Account (HSA). These personal savings accounts are part of Aetna health insurance tax free savings account, whereby individuals can apply a portion of their pretax income towards the account, which can accrue interest, the account and its subsequent generated interest would be utilized for covered or future health care costs. This option is only provided for high deductible Aetna health insurance plans.[8]

There are two types of health care plans within the high deductible PPO. These are the PPO High Deductible 3500 and the PPO High Deductible 5500. Both are HSA compatible.

The PPO High Deductible 3500 has a lower premium and an annual individual deductible of $3500 or $7000 for family. After the deductible has been met, then the enrollee pays only 10% of most covered services, which means that coinsurance is 10% after the deductible has been met.[9]

Coinsurance is similar to copay with the difference that co-pay is a set amount that the insured has to pay for covered services while the insurer pays the rest of the cost of provided service. On the other hand coinsurance is whereby the insurer pays a percentage of the total costs of services provided. With this type of Aetna health plan the co-insurance is 10%. That means that if for example the cost of provided services say diagnostic uterine ultrasound for uterine fibroids is $1500, the insured will pay $150 coinsurance for the ultrasound, which is 10% of the total cost of the ultrasound while the insurer will pay the balance of $1350. If the copay was only $50 for diagnostic tests, then the insured will conversely pay only $50 copay. Thus with coinsurance the insured generally pays more of the health services costs especially when costs of health services are on the increase. It is also important to note that with all Aetna health insurance plans the copay is usually not due at the time the medical service is rendered, but billed separately to the patient and is not applicable towards coinsurance or out of pocket maximum.

Therefore under this particular Aetna health plan the insured will pay 10% coinsurance for office visits, prescriptions, hospitalization, skilled nursing, physical/occupational therapy, and home health care, with out of pocket maximum of $5950 for individual and $11,900 for family within network services. This plan also provides the enrollee the opportunity to see any licensed health care professional within and outside the Aetna network, though the enrollee will pay more out of pocket if they choose to utilize a health care profession that is outside of the Aetna network. This is because Aetna does not have a reduced reimbursement rate contract with out of network health care providers and doctors.[10] For out of network services, the deductible is $10,000 for individuals and $20,000 for family and out of pocket maximum is $12,500 for individual and $25,000 for family. Coinsurance maximum is $2500 for individual and $5000 for family under this plan. Coinsurance after the deductible has been met is 50% for covered services, when utilizing health care services outside of the network. Maternity is not covered for both in network or out network within this plan, except for the rare instances where there are complications. This plan covers generic and preferred brand oral contraceptives but does not cover non preferred brand oral contraceptives and will cover self injectibles with 10% coinsurance for in network but will not cover it for out of network. [11]

The Aetna PPO High Deductible 5500 has a lower premium than PPO High Deductible 3500, but with higher deductible and 0% copay and coinsurance for most covered services. Just like with PPO 3500, this particular plan also provides the enrollee the option of utilizing any licensed health care professional within and outside the Aetna network, though the enrollee will pay more out of pocket if they choose to utilize a health care profession that is outside of the Aetna network. The annual deductible is $5,500 for individual and $11,000 for family, likewise the out of pocket maximum is $5500 for individual and $11,000 for family, within network. After the maximum has been reached, then there is 0% coinsurance, for office visit, prescription drugs, hospitalization, skilled nursing, home health care and physical/occupational therapy.[12] For out of network services, the deductible is $10,000 for individuals and $20,000 for family and out of pocket maximum is $12,500 for individual and $25,000 for family. Coinsurance maximum is $2500 for individual and $5000 for family under this plan. Coinsurance after the deductible has been met is 50% for covered services for out of network utilization. Maternity is also not covered for both in network or out network within this plan, except for the rare instances where there are pregnancy complications. This plan covers generic and both preferred and non-preferred brand oral contraceptives but does not cover self-injectable out of network, though it covers self-injectable within network at 0% coinsurance. [13]

Aetna also offers a PPO plan that allows the enrollee to use any of the "Preferred Providers," including specialists, family doctors and hospitals. Preferred providers are health care providers that have contracted with health insurance companies to offer health care services at a reduced rate. The reduced rates are what the health insurance company will pay them when they render medical services to enrollees within that particular health insurance plan. Thus usually within a health insurance plan, enrollees that utilize the services of preferred providers would not have to pay beyond the stipulated coinsurance or copay whereas if they utilize health care providers outside the plan they would have to pay more out of pocket costs since the health insurance agency does not have the reduced fee agreement with out of network health care providers.

Thus Aetna PPO has a set of benefits provided for utilization of in network providers and another for outside network providers, with enrollees paying more for utilization of outside network providers. Aetna PPO plan provides coverage for specialist care, hospital and emergency care, prescription drugs, outpatient surgery and preventive care such as routine exams and annual physicals. The selection of a Primary Care Physician (PCP) is not required for this type of plan and neither is a referral required in order to see a provider within the network. There are several plans within the PPO, with varying deductibles. [14] There are PPO 1500, PPO 2500, PPO 5000 and PPO 7500 with unlimited primary care visits plus dental.

Aetna PPO 1500 is a preferred provider organization health plan with a lower annual deductible as well as out of pocket maximum but with higher monthly premiums. Just like the other Aethna plans mentioned above this plan also provides the enrollee the opportunity of utilizing any licensed health care professional within and outside the Aetna network, though the enrollee will pay more out of pocket if they choose to utilize a health care profession that is outside of the Aetna network. This health care plan has an annual deductible of $1500 for individuals and $3000 for family, with an out of pocket maximum of $4500 for an individual and $9000 for family and a co-insurance of 20% within network once the deductible has been reached, up until the out of pocket maximum is reached at which point the insurance covers all the costs. There is a $500 prescription drug deductible after which the enrollee pays $15 copay with the deductibles waived for generic drug prescription including oral contraceptive, for both in and out network. The deductible does not apply to generic drugs.

There is $35 copay for preferred drugs including oral contraceptives and $65 copay for non-preferred prescription drugs including oral contraceptives. For out of network preferred brand there is $35 copay plus 50% after deductible has been reached and for non-preferred brand there is $65 copay plus 50% after deductible has been reached. There is 30% coinsurance after the deductible has been reached for self-injectable prescriptions, but that is not covered out of network, for this health care plan. [15] Thus it is much more cost efficient for the enrollee to stay within network and with preferred brand or generic drugs.   Under this plan there is $35 office copay for non-specialist visits and $50 copay for Specialist visits. Then after the deductible has been reached, there is 20% Coinsurance for skilled nursing, hospitalization, home health care and physical/occupational therapy. But if the enrollee has reached the out of pocket maximum the insurance then pays for all the health care costs.[16]

Another health plan option offered by Aetna is PPO 2500, which offers its subscribers a higher monthly premium than PPO 1500, but with lower annual deductible and out of pocket maximum. This health plan also provides the option of utilizing the services of any health care provider both within and outside the network, with of course higher coinsurances/copays for utilizing providers outside of network. The plan has an annual deductible of $2500 for individual and $5000 for family, with out of pocket maximums of $7500 for individual and $15,000 for family within network, while out of network annual deductible is $5000 and $10,000 for individual and family respectively. The coinsurance maximum for out of network is $5000 and $10,000 and out of pocket maximum is $10,000 and $20,000, for individuals and family respectively. Upon reaching the deductible a co-insurance of 20% within network applies, unless the out of pocket maximum is reached at which point the insurance covers all the costs.[309] There is a $500 prescription drug deductible, which is not applicable to generic drugs. Thus the enrollee pays $15 copay for generic drugs in network and out of network pays $15 copay plus 50% of the cost of the prescription. The generic drug deductible waiver is applicable to all prescriptions including oral contraceptives, for both in and out network. There is $35 copay for preferred drugs including oral contraceptives and $65 copay for non-preferred prescription drugs including oral contraceptives. For out of network preferred brand there is $35 copay plus 50% after deductible has been reached and for non-preferred brand there is $65 copay plus 50% after deductible has been reached. There is 30% coinsurance after the deductible has been reached for self- injectibles, but that is not covered out of network, for this health care plan.17 Thus far it can clearly be seen that it is more cost efficient for an enrollee to stay within network and with preferred brand or generic drugs.[18]

Under this plan there is $40 office copay for non-specialist visits and $50 copay for specialist visits in network with the deductibles waived. After the deductible has been reached, there is 20% coinsurance for skilled nursing, hospitalization, home health care and physical/occupational therapy. But if the enrollee has reached the out of pocket maximum the insurance then pays for all the health care costs.[19] F

PPO 5000 is another health plan option offered by Aetna insurance company, that is similar to the above two mentioned plans, except that it offers lower monthly premiums coupled with higher annual deductible and out of pocket amount. The $500 prescription drug deductible is also applicable here, as well as the same $15, $35 and $65 co-pay for generic, preferred and non-preferred drugs respectively. Self-injectibles are covered both for within and out of network at the same rate as for PPO 2500. Annual deductible is $5000 and $10,000 in network for individual and family respectively, and for out of network is $10,000 and $20,000 respectively. Coinsurance maximum is $5000 and $10,000 in network and $2500 and $5000 out of network for individual and family respectively, thus the coinsurance maximum is less out of network than with in network, but there is 20% coinsurance and 50% coinsurance after deductible up to out of pocket maximum for in network and out of network respectively. Therefore once the out of pocket maximum has been realized, the enrollee will pay $0 both within and out of network health care services. Out of pocket maximum is $10,000 and $20,000 for in network and $12,500 and $25,000 for out of network for individual and family respectively. Maternity is not covered for these plans except when there is complication.[20] The rest of this plan coverage mirrors that of PPO 2500 with 20% coinsurance and 50% coinsurance after deductible for in network and out network respectively for most care. There is 40% coinsurance for complex imaging for in network imaging services. There is no copay nor deductible applicable to in network preventive care/routine physical (including lab work and X rays) or annual routine gynecological exams, likewise the copay is $40 and the deductible is waived for non-specialist office visit and the same is applicable to specialist care with $50 copay for in network care and likewise for urgent care with $75 copay. For those services out of network, there is still the usual 50% coinsurance. The $350 Emergency room copay is waived for both in and out of network only if the enrollee is actually admitted.[21]

Another Aetna health plan is PPO 7500 with unlimited Primary Care Visits plus Dental, which provides a lower monthly premium though with a higher annual deductible as well as higher out of pocket maximum amount. Similar to the other health plan options mentioned above the enrollee has the choice of any health care professional and the option of going outside the network for medical service. Individuals enrolled within the plan have $7500 and $15,000 for within network and $10,000 and $20,000 outside network respectively for individual and family deductibles. There is likewise for individual and family respectively, an out of pocket maximum of $10,000/20,000 within network and $12,500/$25,000 for out of network. The co-insurance maximum is $2500/$5000 respectively for individual and family for both within and outside of network. There is a 20% coinsurance within network and 50% coinsurance out of network, after the deductible has been met up to the out of pocket limit.[22]

For in network services and annual routine gynecological exam, the deductible is waived and there is no copay, thought the 50% coinsurance is still applicable for out of network services for those two categories. There is $40 and $50 copay and waiver of deductibles for utilization of within network non specialist office visit as well as for urgent care facility use respectively. Out of network utilization would incur a 50% coinsurance, unless specifically mentioned otherwise.[23]

There is no coverage for self-injectable, preferred and non-preferred prescription drugs under this plan, both for within and out of network. There is a $20 copay and waiver of deductible for generic drug prescription, although for out of network, there is $20 co-pay plus 50% coinsurance on cost of generic drug.[24] Thus technically the high deductible nature of this plan basically guarantees unlimited primary care visits, and can be attractive because it also includes dental coverage.

Aetna also offers PPO value plans, which aim to save money for enrollees. These value plans include PPO value 10000, PPO Value 5000 and Preventive and Hospital care 3000.

The PPO value 10000 has similar plan features with the other PPO plans, except that there is more of a focus on lower monthly premiums with higher out of pocket maximum and yearly deductible. Both in network and out network deductible are the same, $10,000 for individual and $20,000 for family. Out of pocket maximum is the same for both in and out network at $12,500 for individual and $25,000 for family. For PPO value 10000 the coinsurance maximum is $2500 for individual and $5000 for family both for in and out of state network. This health care plan has the deductible waived for within network non specialist office visit and urgent care facility visit but attaches a co-pay of $40 and $75 respectively for such visits. Specialist visits are 20% of service change after the deductible has been reached. Hospital and outpatient surgery are 20% coinsurance after the deductible has been reached. For out of network services on the other hand there is 50% coinsurance for all health care services provided, including for preventive health. Emergency room copay of $500 is waived for both in and out network if admitted. Maternity is not covered for both except if there are complications, but within network, routine gynecological exam is covered without copay and the deductible is waived though for out of network services there is still a 50% coinsurance.

Under this plan there is no deductible for pharmacy, though there is no coverage for both preferred and non-preferred brand drugs and for self injectibles for both in and out network, only generic is covered. Generic oral contraceptive is covered at $20 copay for in network. For out of network pharmacies, generic oral contraceptives are covered for at $20 copay plus 50% coinsurance, the deductible is waived for both.[25] Therefore this plan as well as the other Aethna health care plans shows that, despite the fact that individuals have the option of going out of network for their healthcare services, it is much more expensive than staying in network to receive such services.

PPO Value 5000, plan combines higher annual deductibles and out of pocket maximum with lower monthly premium and the autonomy of utilizing the services of any licensed health care professional within the Aetna or outside Aetna network for covered services. Just like with the other aforementioned plans, utilization of out of network services are usually accompanied by higher deductibles and co-payments. In network deductible is $5000 for individuals and $10,000 for family, with 20%/40% coinsurance once the deductible has been met, while out network deductible is $10,000 for individual and $20,000 for family, with 50% coinsurance when the deductible has been met. Co-insurance maximum is $5000/$10,000 for individual and family respectively within network and $2500/$5000 for individual and family respectively for out of network services. At the same time, out of pocket maximum is less for within network than outside of network at $10,000/$20,000 individual and family respectively for in network services versus $12,500/$25,000 individual and family respectively for out of network services.[26]

This health care plan has the deductible waived for within network non specialist office visit and urgent care facility visit but attaches copays of $40 and $75 respectively for such visits. Specialist visits are 20% of service charge after the deductible has been reached, just like in PPO value 10000. Annual routine gynecological exams have $0 copay and the deductible is waived for in network services, But hospital and outpatient surgery are 40% coinsurance after the deductible has been reached. For out of network services on the other hand, there is 50% coinsurance for all health care services provided, including for preventive health and routine gynecological exams.

Emergency room copay of $500 is waived for both in and out network if admitted. Maternity is not covered for both except if there are complications. Under this plan, only generic pharmaceuticals are covered and the deductible is waived for both in and out network, with only a $20 copay.[27] Therefore this plan is somewhat similar to the PPO value 10000 with minor differences, and it is still much more expensive going out of network for healthcare services than staying within network to receive such services.

The final health insurance plan provided by Aetna for Tennessee residents is Preventive and Hospital Care 3000 or HSA compatible. It is known as HSA compatible because there is the possibility or option of opening a tax-advantaged Health Savings Account (HSA) if desired. A HSA is part of a health plan whereby an enrollee will deposit money into a specific account. The deposited funds are tax sheltered and could be saved to be utilized for future health care costs or used immediately to pay for covered health care services. If the money is saved for future health care expenses, they would be accumulating interest within the account. It is important to note that, in order to be eligible for a HSA, an enrollee must have high deductible health insurance plan.[28]

Thus with this plan, not only is there the option of having a HSA, there is also lower annual deductible and out of pocket maximum as well as a lower monthly premium. There is a focus within this plan on utilizing preventive care so as to avoid more expensive medical complications down the road. And just like with other Aetna plans there is the autonomy to utilize the services of any licensed health care provider for health care services, both within and outside the network, although it is more expensive to see a health services provider that is outside the Aetna health work. Therefore within this particular plan, network deductible is $3000 for individuals and $6,000 for family, with 20% coinsurance once the deductible has been met, up until the out of pocket maximum is reached, then it is $0 coinsurance for the rest of the year. Out of network deductible is $6,000 for individual and $12,000 for family, with 50% coinsurance when the deductible has been met, up until the out of pocket maximum is reached. Co-insurance maximum is $2000/$4,000 for individual and family respectively within network and $4000/$8000 for individual and family respectively for out of network services. Out of pocket maximum is more for out of network than within network health care services. The out of pocket maximum is at $5,000/$10,000 for individual and family respectively for in network services versus $10000/$20,000 for individual and family respectively for out of network services.[29]

This plan does not cover quite a range of medical services, regardless of whether in network or outside network. The services that are not covered include pharmacy, non-specialist office visit, specialist visit, urgent care facility, non-preventive lab/x-ray, or complex imaging as well as durable medical equipment and physical occupational therapy. But under this plan, for in network services, annual routine gynecological exams and preventive health/routine physicals are covered with $0 copay and waived deductibles. On the other hand, skilled nursing, home health care, outpatient surgery and hospital admissions are covered at 20% after the deductible has been reached, and for out of network health care services covered by this plan, the co-pay is 50% of charges after the deductible has been reached.[30] Invariably the focus of this particular health insurance plan is on providing preventive and hospital care as the name implies.

Another insurance company that provides health insurance services in Tennessee is Blue Cross Blue shield of Tennessee. This health insurance company provides comprehensive differing plans as well for Tennessee residents and nationwide, and the plans range from High Deductible Health Savings Account (HAS) compatible plans to differing Preferred Provider organizations (PPO) plans with different ranges of deductibles. BlueCross BlueShield also provides short term health plans to individuals that qualify.

Connecticut General Life Insurance (CIGNA) is another major provider of health insurance coverage within Tennessee as well as nationwide. This organization is a huge health insurance company that operates within USA as well as internationally within 30 countries. It is also a component of the S&P 500 and is listed with the New York Stock Exchange (NYSE: CI) and is a component of the S&P 500 stock index. Cigna, just like BlueCross BlueShield and Aetna, provide comprehensive differing plans as well for Tennessee residents.

Apart from Aetna, BlueCross BlueShield, Cigna, there are twelve other companies that provide health insurance coverage in Tennessee namely, American Republic Insurance, Celtic Insurance, Coventry health and Life Insurance, Freedom life Insurance Company of America, Golden Rule Insurance Company, Guarantee Trust Life Insurance, Humana Insurance, Independence American Insurance, MEGA life and Health Insurance, National Foundation Life Insurance, Assurant Insurance and World Insurance companies. All these insurance companies provide a varied range of health insurance protection but the underlying criteria is that all of these insurance companies that operate within Tennessee have to adhere to the applicable tenants of the Patient Protection and Affordable care Act. A lot of them have made strides in conforming to the requirements of the federal health care law, including increasing the age for eligible dependable children to 26 years as well as having no life time limits on coverage. It would be interesting to see how the health care companies adapt when the bulk of the mandates of the health care law take effect in 2014.

1. Aexcel designated specialists are Specialist doctors within the Aetna health care plan or network whom are considered to have met industry wide nationally recognized accepted practices for clinical performance as well as meeting Aetna's efficiency Standards.
2 . Aetna Facts. (n.d.). Retrieved September 3, 2012, from Aetna.com: http://www.aetna.com/about-aetna-insurance/aetna-corporate-profile/facts.html
3. Ibid
4 . Understanding Aexcel. (n.d.). Retrieved September 3, 2012, from Aetna.com: http://www.aetna.com/plans-services-health-insurance/detail/assets/documents/Member-brochure.pdf
5. Ibid
6. Ibid
7. Aetna Tennessee Health Insurance Plan Choices. (n.d.). Retrieved September 3, 2012, from http://healthinsurance.aetna.com/state/tennessee/individual-health-insurance/health-plans.
8. Ibid
9. Ibid
10. Ibid
11. Take Charge of Your Health. (n.d.). Retrieved September 3, 2012, from Aetna: http://healthinsurance.aetna.com/media/pdf_plans/TN_Direct.pdf
12. Aetna Tennessee Health Insurance Plan Choices
13. Take Charge of Your Health
14. Aetna Tennessee Health Insurance Plan Choices
15. Take Charge of Your Health
16. Ibid
17. Ibid
18. Ibid
19. Aetna Tennessee Health Insurance Plan Choices
20. Take Charge of Your Health
21. Ibid
22. Ibid
23. Ibid
24. Ibid
25. Ibid
26. Ibid
27. Ibid
28. Aetna Tennessee Health Insurance Plan Choices
29. Ibid
30. Ibid

Chapter 7

Impact of Affordable Care Act on Insurance Companies

President Obama won reelection on November 6th 2012, thereby assuring that his health care reform plan would not be overturned. His opponent former Massachusetts Governor, Mitt Romney broadly campaigned on overturning the Patient Protection and Affordable Care Act. But since the republican presidential contender Mitt Romney did not win the election, there is now the assured possibility that the main tenants or requirements of the health reform plan will fully go into effect during reelected President Obama's second 4 year term. This is especially true since the Supreme Court has upheld the main fundamentals of the federal health care reform law. Several main provisions of the health reform plan will go into effect in 2014 during the course of President Obama's second term.

Since President Obama's, reelection, there has been marked effort at ensuring that the main provisions of the Affordable Care Act would now be implemented. The health reform act was predicated on the expansion of health insurance coverage to about 32 million individuals whom were previously uninsured.[1] Inherent in achieving this goal, is the expansion of Medicaid, as well as the individual mandate which requires people to buy health insurance and the additional incentives to employers to provide health care insurance for their employees. The totality of these measures would help bring about an additional 32 million individuals within the health insured fold.

An overview of some of the key regulations of Patient Protection and Affordable Care Act, that would be phased in during President Obama's second term in office.

Essential Health Benefits

The Health Care reform plan delineates some health insurance benefits as being essential and mandatory to any health insurance plan or provision. As such, those benefits must be covered by health insurance plans of all sizes, including both self-funded and fully insured group coverage. Also starting on or after January 1 2014, there would be no lifetime maximums or annual dollar limits by group health plans on such essential health benefits and pharmacy benefits for both in network and out of network services, but the reform does not necessarily exclude plan limits on number of health care visits.

According to United health care, "Annual limits may not be less than the following amounts.

"For plan years beginning before Jan. 1, 2014:

- $750,000 on or after Sept. 23, 2010
- $1.25 million on or after Sept. 23, 2011
- $2 million on or after Sept. 23, 2012 to Jan. 1, 2014.[2]
- Grandfathered Group health plans and group health insurance coverage are still expected to abide by the non-annual limits mandate for EHB. It is important to mention that as applicable by law, insurance plans may impose annual limits on non-essential Health Benefits. The following provisions are categorized by the reform plan as Essential Health Benefits (EHB):
  o Hospitalization
  o Ambulatory patient services
  o Emergency services
  o Maternity and newborn care
  o Pediatric services, including oral and vision care
  o Laboratory services
  o Mental health and substance abuse disorder services (including behavioral health treatment)
  o Prescription drugs
  o Preventive and wellness services and chronic disease management
  o Rehabilitative and facilitative services and devices."[3]

Therefore, starting from January, 2014, fully insured individual and small group markets, with non-grandfathered plans, both outside and within health insurance exchanges, Medicaid benchmark, and benchmark equivalent as well as Basic Health Programs must cover the EHB. According to the Department of Health and Human Services this is structured so as to balance affordability, comprehensiveness and state flexibility during the process of development of Essential Health benefits. Thus each state has to select a current health plan as a "benchmark" or standard, to be utilized in the establishment of items and services that would be included within the Essential Health Benefits package for 2014-2015. The states have the opportunity to choose as a benchmark from one of four health insurance plan options. If the state neglects to choose or set a benchmark then by default their benchmark will automatically be the small group plan with the largest enrollment within that particular state. Generally states define "Small group" plans as insurance provided to an employer that has 50 or less employees. Starting from 2014, the states have the opportunity to raise that number of employees that constitute a small group plan to 100. But the standard number within a small group plan, starting from 2016, would be defined as having 1-100 employees, within that particular health plan. The Department of Health and Human Services (HHS) would reassess the proposed benchmark for the period spanning 2016 and beyond, but the current benchmark process would be effective for the period 2014 up to 2016. The health plan options that could be selected as a benchmark are as follows:

Any of the below plans could be chosen as a benchmark:

- The three largest federal employee health plan options;
- The three largest state employee health plans;
- The largest HMO plan offered within the state's commercial market
- The largest plan based on enrollment in any of the three largest small group products within the state.[4]

It is important to note that according to HHS, the obligation to cover the essential health benefits is not mandated upon self-insured group health plans, health coverage offered within the large group market and grandfathered health plans. [5]

Health Insurance Exchanges

The Health Care Reform Act stipulates that states have until January 1, 2013, to be approved by the Department of Health and Human Services, for their individual state exchanges. Once a particular state has been approved that means it now has the certification to provide exchanges within their individual state. Those states that win the approval for state exchanges must be available for enrollment starting from mid-2013. Thus by 2014, states are required to have set up Health Insurance Exchanges. These health insurance exchanges are supposed to make it easier for individuals or small businesses to purchase health insurance. If a state opts out of providing health insurance exchanges, then the state's residents can purchase insurance through the federal government exchanges. By January 1 of 2015, the exchanges should be financially self-sufficient and by January 1, of 2017, the state exchanges may then be open to large employers. As of December 18, 2012, 18 states and the District of Columbia had indicated that they intend to run their own health insurance exchanges. Seven other states will operate exchanges in federal state partnership exchanges. Therefore within the 25 states that did not submit blueprint for running their own health care exchanges, the federal government will implement federal health insurance exchanges within those particular states.

The state health exchanges were a key indication of the Affordable Care Act, in that uninsured state residents and small businesses could accesses their state's exchange website and compare prices on health insurance plans and options prior to buying health insurance for themselves.

There was a lot of initial opposition to President Obama's health care reform plan, with a lot of republican governors showing a lot of resistance to applying for state exchanges. Thus, as of Dec 18, 2012, only five republican Governor led states have indicated that they would run their own health care exchanges and another two republican Governor led states will run a federal state partnership exchange, despite the fact that the Department of Health and Human Services has awarded about $314 million in grants to help states towards the formation of state health exchanges. With regards to choice and scope of coverage there is no expectation that the state led health insurance exchanges would be vastly different from the federal health insurance exchanges. But the idea behind having state health insurance exchanges is that states would be better able to tailor health plan options to better accommodate the particular needs of their residents and their Medicaid populations. There would be four levels or four types of health insurance plans within the exchanges, based on the level of health coverage they provide. The four levels of plans are namely bronze, silver, gold and platinum, with the bronze providing the most basic and least comprehensive of plans and the platinum providing the most comprehensive of coverage.

About 30 million uninsured individuals are expected to be helped by the health care reform, which is designed to expand Medicaid as well as help create subsidies for lower income individuals to utilize in buying private insurance. The establishment of the exchanges is to help facilitate that. The Department of Health and Human Services project that about 25 million individuals are expected to utilize the health insurance exchanges, and out of that number about 19 million would probably be eligible for federal premium assistance tax credit. The Affordable Care Act mandates that from January 2014, individuals that purchase their health insurance through exchanges would be eligible for health insurance premium subsidies as well as cost sharing, if their income is less than 400% of the Federal Poverty level, or $89,000 for a family of four, as of 2011.

Low income individuals with employer insurance that have high premiums (more than 9.5% of their household income) or inadequate plans (plans that pay less than 60% of covered benefits) can go to the exchanges for subsidized insurance.[6] There are two different types of subsidies provided by the Affordable Care Act.

Type 1:

There is the monthly premium assistance tax credit, which basically means that an individual or family could go ahead and apply for the tax credit after buying and maintaining health insurance for which they pay a monthly fee. It must be noted that the individuals that qualify have the option of applying for the tax credit. This they can do regardless of if their state operates a state health insurance exchange or is in a state/federal insurance exchange partnership or if their resident state is part of a federal administered insurance exchange.

The qualified individuals do not have to apply for the monthly premium assistance tax credit if they do not wish to do so. The premium assistances are only available through the health insurance exchanges, and are determined on an income based sliding basis, thus the less income one makes, the more the subsidized help. Such subsidies are based on the premium for the second lowest cost plan or silver plan, thus if an individual or family wants a higher cost or higher tier health insurance plan (that is gold or platinum), they would have to pay the difference.[7] Regardless of if individuals file their taxes or not they would still be eligible for credits if they meet the requirements. These credits would be paid directly in advance to the chosen insurer, but the individual would be responsible for the balance premium, that way people would not have to pay their premiums and then wait for their reimbursement to be sent to them.

It is also important to note, that within states that have federally facilitated exchanges, there is a tax assessment for large employers with 50 or more employees that do not provide affordable employer health insurance for their employees, thus causing such employees to seek health insurance through the state or federal health insurance exchanges. In order for the employer tax assessment to occur, the employees that got their insurance through the health insurance exchange, must be eligible and have applied for the premium assistance tax credit, which helps reduce the premium amount that they pay.

Table 7.1- Premium Limits for Consumers Based on Income

Income	Premium Limit
Up to 133% FPL	2% of income
133 - 150% FPL	3 - 4% of income
150 - 200% FPL	4 - 6.3% of income
200 - 250% FPL	6.3 - 8.05% of income
250 - 300% FPL	8.05 - 9.5% of income
350 - 400% FPL	9.5% of income

Premium Limits for Consumers.[8]

Type 2:

Then, there is cost sharing assistance, which helps reduce the amount of maximum out of pocket payments that an insured individual will make to a health care provider. It is important to note that all individuals that buy insurance through health insurance exchanges will have a cap or limit on their out of pocket expenses, which would include deductibles, coinsurance and copayments. Usually premium credits allow people to buy silver insurance plan through the exchange. The silver plan has an actuarial value of 70, meaning that the plan covers about 70% of the total cost of care and the insured person has to cover the remaining 30% cost of care. However, individuals that are at or below 250% of the federal poverty level will receive cost sharing assistance, with the end result that they would not pay the balance 30% of their silver plan. As such, if the individual is at or below 250% of the federal poverty level, which is an income of about $55,000 for a family of four, then that particular individual would receive cost sharing credits. These cost sharing credits will reduce out of pocket expenses as well as reduce other cost sharing expenses such as deductibles, co-payments and coinsurance.[9]

The cost sharing mechanism, thereby ensures that the lower the income level the higher the actuarial value of the insurance plan enrolled in, simply because the 30% coinsurance is offset by the cost sharing which is based or determined by income level. Thus an individual that is below 150% of the federal poverty level would be enrolled in a silver plan but with the offsetting cost sharing will have a health insurance with an actuarial value of about 94%. That means that the individual's coinsurance would effectively be capped at 6%. This is to insure that individuals can still afford to see health care providers when they need to for their health well-being.

The capping of the out of pocket limits is modeled after those limits that are applicable to high deductible plans used with Health Savings Accounts. So effectively those below the Federal poverty level get subsidies to lower the cap rate on their health plan's coinsurance.

Table 7.2- Out of Pocket Spending Limits for Consumers Based on Income [10]

Income	Out-of-Pocket Limit (based on 2011 HSA limit)
100 - 200% FPL	1/3 HSA limit ($1,983/individual; $3,967/family)
200 - 300% FPL	1/2 HSA limit ($2,975/individual; $5,950/family)
300 - 400% FPL	2/3 HSA ($3,967/individual; $7,933/family)
Above 400% FPL	100% HSA limit ($5,950/individual; $11,500/family)

*low-income individuals and families will be able to enroll in health plans with lower deductibles and co-payments.

Table 7.3- Actuarial Value of Coverage Base on Income [11]

Percentage of poverty line	Income	Percentage of Income	Monthly dollar amount	Actuarial value of coverage
Family of four:				
133 - 150%	$29,547 - $33,075	3 - 4%	$74 - $110	94%
150 - 200%	$33,075 - $44,100	4 - 6.3%	$110 - $232	87%
200 - 250%	$44,100 - $55,125	6.3 - 8.1%	$232 - $372	73%
250 - 300%	$55,125 - $66,150	8.1 - 9.5%	$372 - $524	70%
300 - 350%	$66,150 - $77,175	9.5%	$524 - $611	70%
350 - 400%	$77,175 - $88,200	9.5%	$611 - $698	70%
Individual:				
133 - 150%	$14,512 - $16,245	3-4%	$36 - $54	94%
150 - 200%	$16,245 - $21,660	4-6.3%	$54 - $114	87%
200 - 250%	$21,660 - $27,075	6.3-8.1%	$114 - $182	73%
250 - 300%	$27,075 - $32,490	8.1-9.5%	$182 - $257	70%
300 - 350%	$32,490 - $37,905	9.5%	$257 - $300	70%
350 - 400%	$37,905 - $43,320	9.5%	$300 - $343	70%

*Note the 30% is average for the beneficial population that does not mean that every individual's initial cost sharing would be set at 30%.

Grandfathered Plans

Under the Affordable Care Act, a grandfathered plan is a group health insurance policy or plan that was in place, prior to and up to the enactment of the Patient Protection and Affordable Care Act, on March 23rd 2010. The plan must have provided continual coverage up to the March 23rd 2010 date. Grand fathered plans are exempt from some of the requirements of PPACA. Health plans are considered grandfathered unless employers make changes to coverage or requirements of the health plans. Such changes would include reducing the provision of benefits, any increase in member coinsurance, or reduction in the amount paid towards benefits coverage for employees by more than 5%, (usually resulting in increased employee payment share of the cost of the plan), increasing copays and deductibles and out of pocket limits by amounts not allowed by the reform plan. If such a scenario occurs then the plan will lose its grandfathered status. Any coverage or benefits changes made by grandfathered plans are compared to the benefits in place by March 23rd 2010, in making the determination if grandfathered status is lost. That helps determine if the reduction of benefits occurred after March 23, 2010, when the health care law was passed. But generally grandfathered plans do not lose their grandfathered status if employers switch plan funding from self-insured to fully funded or if they change insurance companies to other companies that offer similar benefits provisions, or if they take in more members or increase their plan benefits. But if an enrollee is a member of a grandfathered plan then some of the requirements of PPACA may not be applicable to that particular enrollee, regardless, that enrollee may see new additional benefits as the grandfathered plan complies with applicable provisions of PPACA.

Therefore, grandfathered plans are still required to comply with some of the provisions of PPACA. For instance if a grandfathered plan offers dependent coverage, then such coverage must extend to dependents up to 26 years of age, although until 2014, grandfathered plans may exclude adult dependents that are eligible for other group health insurance plans coverage through their jobs. Also grandfathered plans cannot exclude potential enrollees under the age of 19 because they have preexisting conditions and they cannot have lifetime coverage limit on services deemed essential health benefits by PPACA.

The law does not likewise mandate that grandfathered plans must provide preventive care without cost sharing from enrollees, therefore grandfathered plans may keep the same preventive health plans they had prior to or on 23rd March 2010. For instance non-grandfathered plans that do not have a religious exemption, are required by the new law, starting from August 1, 2012, to provide additional preventive care services including contraceptives for women without any cost sharing. Grandfather health care plans do not have to do that.

Another key regulation component of PPACA is the individual mandate as discussed earlier: Under the requirements of the individual mandate, starting from January 1, 2014, all adults must have minimum essential health insurance coverage, otherwise known as Minimum Essential Coverage (MEC). A person may garner health insurance coverage from on or off the insurance exchanges that will be available starting from January 1 2014. For the purposes of the Act, a person has MEC, if they have an individual plan, or a government sponsored health plan or employer sponsored plan. According to Cigna, "If a person cannot keep minimum essential coverage, the Internal Revenue Service will collect a tax penalty from him or her. The monthly tax penalty is described as 1/12th of the greater of:

- For 2014: $95 per uninsured adult in the household (capped at $285 per household) or one percent of the household income over the filing threshold
- For 2015: $325 per uninsured adult in the household (capped at $975 per household) or two percent of the household income over the filing threshold
- For 2016: $695 per uninsured adult in the household (capped at $2,085 per household) or 2.5 percent of the household income over the filing threshold

The penalty will be half of the amount for people under age 18.
There are a few exceptions to the penalty, including:

- Religious reasons
- Not present in the United States
- In prison
- Not able to pay for coverage that is more than eight percent of the household income
- An income that is below 100 percent of the poverty Level
- Having a hardship waiver
- Not covered for less than three months during the year."[12]

Therefore, the tax penalties, though seemingly minimal are supposed to act as a deterrent for those who would normally forgo getting health insurance coverage. And as mentioned earlier, for those individuals that it would present a great fiscal burden to purchase health insurance, there is the possibility of federal premium assistance. The individual mandate aspect of the health insurance reform as discussed in an earlier chapter was one of the basis of challenge of PPACA, but the United States Supreme Court found that mandate constitutional.

Guaranteed Issue and Renewal and Rescissions

Prior to the enactment of PPACA, health insurers may deny issuing a policy to an individual health insurance applicant because that applicant had utilized extensive health care services the prior year or because that individual had an existing condition. Another major component of PPACA, involves the concept or idea that under the health reform plan, insurers must issue a health plan to any individual or group that applies for health coverage regardless of their health conditions or other factors. This is known as the concept of guaranteed issue. Therefore, starting from January 1, 2014, insurers may not deny coverage to an individual because of pre-existing conditions, nor exclude coverage of certain conditions because of preexisting condition. Insurers are also not allowed to charge higher individual premiums based on the health status of the health insurance applicant nor charge higher premiums of small employers (those with 50 or less employees), but this protection does not specifically apply to large employers. It must also be noted that as of September, 2010, insurers in the individual market cannot deny coverage to children under 19 years of age because of pre-existing condition, this protection extends to adults over 19 years of age on January 1, 2014. Also, under the concept of guaranteed renewal, a health insurer may not deny the renewal of an individual or group policy based on high incidence of health care usage, by the individual or group during the prior year. But health insurers may decide not to renew health insurance policy for any of the reasons mentioned below, without running a breach of PPACA:

- "If the insurer stops offering a type of plan altogether, but the insurer must provide all customers under the canceled plan a chance to buy another
- If premiums are not paid at all, or if they are not paid on time
- In case of fraud by the covered individual or group
- If the consumer moves out of the insurer's geographic service area
- If not enough of a small employers' workers not agree to participate in the plan
- If a small employer does not pay a minimum share of its workers' premiums
- An insurer may discontinue offering all of its coverage in the individual, small group, or large group markets. If so, they must notify state officials and enrollees at least 180 days in advance. The insurer must discontinue and not renew all coverage in one or more markets and may not re-enter that market for five years."[13]

Thus guaranteed issue ensures that any individual that so desired would be able to buy health insurance, and that health insurance would cover the stipulated essential health benefits outlined by the Patient Protection and Affordable Care Act.

Prior to enactment of PPACA, if an insured person got sick, or he/she or the employer made an honest mistake while filing out the health insurance application paperwork, the insurance company could and sometimes did, rescind the sick person's health insurance policy, leaving the individual to bear the costs of thousands of dollars in unpaid insurance claims. A rescission is a retroactive termination of a person's health policy that dates back to when the policy was acquired, thus if a health policy was issued on January of 2012, without the protections of PPACA, the health insurance company could cancel the plan in say November of 2012 and thus refuse to pay all prior covered medical bills that were incurred during the period spanning January 2012 to November 2012. This would leave the individual whose health policy was rescinded to cover the totality of medical costs incurred during that period. The health care reform plan outlaws this practice and precludes all health insurance plans including grandfathered ones from this practice. Therefore an insurance plan cannot cancel or rescind a health insurance policy once a person is covered under the health care plan unless the person intentionally misrepresented a material fact when filing out the application form. This would constitute fraud and be a basis for rescinding the health policy. In the event that a health plan has to cancel a policy for any allowable reason, the law specifies that the health plan should provide a minimum of 30 days written notice to the enrollee and also include information, letting the enrollee know that he/she has a right to appeal the recession decision.[14]

Summary of Benefits and Coverage

Finally, the health care reform law requires that health insurers should provide to all applicants and enrollees a uniform summary of benefits and coverage. As such, starting from February 2012, health insurance companies should have plan and benefits documents that include the following;

- "Four-page overview of plan benefits, cost sharing and limitations
- Required set of examples of how the plan works
- Phone number and internet address for obtaining copies of plan documents
- A Standard glossary of medical and insurance terms must also be available."[15]

This is so as to ensure that applicants and enrollees of the different health insurance plans are cognizant of the benefits they would be getting from each plan, and are clear as to what each plan would cover. Insurance plans that purposefully do not comply with this mandate will be fined $1000 for each enrollee within that particular plan. Thus if there are 20,000 enrollees within that plan they would be fined $20,000,000. That is an appreciable fine for non-compliance.

---

1. Health Insurance 101, ACA Provisions. (n.d.). Retrieved December 29, 2012, from Community Catalyst: http://101.communitycatalyst.org/aca_provisions/aca_basics

2 . Timeline of Provisions. (n.d.). Retrieved December 16, 2012, from UnitedHealthcare:http://www.uhc.com/united_for_reform_resource_center/health_reform_provisi ons/essential_health_benefits.htm
3. Ibid
4 . Essential Health Benefits. (n.d.). Retrieved December 17, 2012, from Cigna: http://www.cigna.com/aboutcigna/informed-on-reform/essential-health-benefits.html
5. Essential Health Benefits Bulletin. (2011, December 16). Retrieved December 17, 2012, from Center for Consumer Information and Insurance Oversight: http://www.uhc.com/live/uhc_com/Assets/Documents/Essential_health_benefits_bulletin. pdf
6. Health Insurance 101. (2011). Retrieved December 19, 2012, from Community Catalyst and Georgetown University Health Policy Institute: http://101.community catalyst.org/aca_provisions/subsidies
7. Ibid
8. Ibid
9. Ibid
10. Ibid
11. Ibid
12. Individual Mandate in Reform. (n.d.). Retrieved December 23, 2012, from Cigna: http://www.cigna.com/aboutcigna/informed-on-reform/individual-mandate.html
13. Health Insurance 101, Key Regulation Concepts. (n.d.). Retrieved Decmeber 29, 2012, from Community Catalyst: http://101.communitycatalyst.org/key_regulation_ concepts?id=0001
14. Health Insurance 101, Rescissions. (n.d.). Retrieved December 29, 2012, from Community Catalyst: http://101.communitycatalyst.org/aca_provisions/consumer_ protections?id=0004
15 Summary of Benefits and Coverage. (n.d.). Retrieved December 29, 2012, from Cigna: http://www.cigna.com/aboutcigna/informed-on-reform/summary-of-benefits-and-coverage.html

Chapter 8

Conclusions

The Patient Protection and Affordable Care Act commonly called ObamaCare was a very ambitious federal health care reform law that was signed into effect on March 10, 2010 by President Barak Obama. Central to the health reform plan was the individual Mandate which ensures that every adult with few exceptions would be required to purchase and maintain health insurance coverage. The mandate was necessary to avoid adverse selection, whereby people buy health insurance only when they become sick. Prior to the health reform, health insurance companies usually precluded adverse selection from occurring by denying coverage to individuals with pre-existing condition. The overarching goal of the health reform plan is for healthy people, not just sick people to buy health insurance. It cannot be overemphasized that health insurance companies could not fiscally survive if only sick people buy insurance. Thus it is necessary to have a large pool of individuals both healthy and sick people within an insurance plan so as to spread the risk. The health care reform plan was predicated on the idea that the individual mandate was necessary in order for the Patient Protection and Affordable Care Act to be viable. Despite the legal challenges mounted against the health reform Act, the Supreme Court ultimately ruled that the health reform as well as the individual mandate was constitutional.

Once the issue of the constitutionality of the reform plan was settled, then the next question that needed to be addressed was whether the reform plan would be able to hold if President Obama did not win reelection, especially since Mitt Romney, the 2012 republican presidential contender and challenger of President Obama to the USA Presidency had campaigned on the promise to repeal "ObamaCare." But that question, did not arise since President Obama won a definitive second term victory, in November of 2012. As such, the main tenants of the health care reform act will take effect during President Obama's second term in office.

There are various aspects or goals of the health reform, chief amongst them, being the expansion of insurance coverage to the previously uninsured or under insured and simultaneous expected cost saving from efficiency and streamlining of delivery of medical services. Some of the tenets of the reform plan, such as expansion of dependent coverage up until age 26, elimination of lifetime benefits, cap limits are already in place but it would take a few years when all the stipulations of the reform plan are in place, to actually evaluate the health care reform to see how successful it is or has been in achieving its broad goals of expanding insurance coverage and benefits while simultaneously trying to keep health care costs down.

Thus far health insurance companies have been doing their best to adjust to the requirements of the health reform mandate. A review of the health insurance companies that provide health insurance in Tennessee indicate that they are thus far in compliance with the stipulations of the Act. It would take some years before the full effects on the reform plan would be felt both within the populace and fiscally within insurance companies and exchanges, but early indicia of some of the tenets of the reform plan point to general acceptance of some of the early mandates, such as expansion of dependent coverage to age 26, elimination of the donut hole and elimination of lifetime cap of benefits. Ultimately, as the full effects of the Act are implemented, then it might be necessary to revisit and reevaluate the Patient Protection and Affordable Care Act and its implementation. Only then could, any conclusive indicia be reached as to its effects and whether policy wise some substantive aspects of the health care reform law need to be reformulated or amended to better serve the policy goals of its implementation.

Bibliography

1115 Waiver Amendment Application. (2002, May 21). State of Oregon.

A Comparative Analysis of 29 Countries. (1998). *OECD Health Data*. Paris: Organization for Economic Cooperation and Development.

A Health Insurance Overview. (n.d.). Retrieved January 2, 2013, from Health Insurance 101: The Basics: http://101.community catalyst.org/basics/overview

A More Secure Future: What the New Healt Law Means for You and Your Family. (n.d.). Retrieved July 23, 2012, from The White House: http://www.whitehouse.gov/healthreform/healthcare-overview#consumer-rights

Abelson, R. (2009, June 30). *Insured but Bankrupted by Health Crisis*. Retrieved August 10, 2012, from The New York Times: http://www.nytimes.com/2009/07/01/business/01meddebt.html?_r=1#

Aetna Facts. (n.d.). Retrieved September 3, 2012, from Aetna.com: http://www.aetna.com/about-aetna-insurance/aetna-corporate-profile/facts.html

Aetna Tennessee Health Insurance Plan Choices. (n.d.). Retrieved September 3, 2012, from http://healthinsurance.aetna.com/ state/tennessee/individual-health-insurance/health-plans

Ahmar, A. R. (n.d.). *How to Defend ObamaCare*. Retrieved July 21, 2012, from Slate: http://www.slate.com/articles/news_and_politics/jurisprudence/2012/03/supreme_court_and_ObamaCare_what_donald_verrilli_should_have_said_to_the_court_s_conservative_justices_.html

Altman, D., & Dennis, B. (1990). Perspectives on the Medicaid Program. *Health Care Financing Review 12*, 2-5.

Balz, D., & Cohen, J. (2009, October 20). *Most Support Public Option for Health Insurance, Poll finds*. Retrieved July 17, 2012, from Washington Post: http://www.washingtonpost.com/wp-dyn/content/article/2009/10/19/AR2009101902451.html

Blum, J. (2012, August 9). *What is the Donut Hole?* Retrieved July 27, 2012, from HealthCare.gov: http://www.healthcare.gov/blog/ 2010/08/donuthole.html

Bodenhimer, T., & Grumbach, K. (1995). The Reconfiguration of US Medicine. *The Journal of the American Medical Association 274 no. 1*, 85-92.

Bonneyman, G. (1996). *Status of TennCare*. Nashville: Center for Health Care Strategies.

Brown, L. (1991). The National Politics of Oregon's Rationing Plan. *Health Affairs 10, no. 2*, 28-51.

Capo. (2009, October 15). *Florida Bonanno Crime Family Members Admit Guilt*. Retrieved July 29, 2012, from Mafiatoday.com: http://mafiatoday.com/bonanno-family/florida-bonanno-crime-family-members-admit-guilt/

CBO Releases Updated Estimates for the Insurance Coverage Provisions of the Affordable Care Act. (2012, March 13). Retrieved August 3, 2012, from Congressional Budget Office: http://www.cbo.gov/ publication/43080

CBO's 2011 Long-term Budget Outlook. (2011, June 22). Retrieved July 13, 2012, from CBO: http://cbo.gov/publication/41486

Center for Medicare and Medicaid Services. (2012, July 24). Retrieved   July 30, 2012, from CMS.gov: http://innovations.cms.gov/

Chase, C. (1998). Changing State and Federal Payment Policies for Medicaid Disproportionate-Share Hospitals. *Health Affairs*.

Children's Pre-existing Conditions. (2012, July 23). Retrieved July 23,   2012,   from HealthCare.gov: http://www.healthcare.gov/law/ features/rights/childrens-pre-existing-conditions/index.html

Cleverly, W. (1978). *Essentials of Health Care Finance*. Rockville, Maryland: Aspen Systems Corporation.

Conis, E., & Medlin, C. (2008, November). *Update on Oregon Health Plan (OHP) Restructuring*.   Retrieved   August   12,   2012,   from http://hpm.org/en/Surveys/IGH_-_USA/11/Update_on_Oregon_ Health_Plan_%28OHP%29_Restructuring.html

Commonwealth Care. (2012). Retrieved August 15, 2012, from MassResources.org: http://www.massresources.org/ commonwealth-care.html#incomelimits

Coordinated Care Organizations. (n.d.). Retrieved August 13, 2012, from Oregon.gov: http://cms.oregon.gov/oha/ohpb/pages/health-reform/ccos.aspx

Coughlin, T., & Liska, D. (1997). The Medicaid Disproportionate Share Hospital Payment Program$: Background and Issues. *The Urban Institute, no. A-14*.

Coughlin, T., & Liska, D. (1999). The Medicaid Disproportionate Share Hospital Payment Program: Background and Issues. *The Urban Institute*.

Covering Young Adults Through Their Parent's of Guardian's Health Policy.   (2012, June). Retrieved July 24, 2012, from National   Conference of State Legislators: http://www.ncsl.org/issues-research/health/   dependent-health-coverage-state-implementation.aspx#State_Actions

Creating a New Competitive Marketplace: Affordable Insurance Exchanges.   (2012, May   16).   Retrieved   July   25,   2012,   from   HealthCare.gov: http://www.healthcare.gov/news/factsheets/2011/05/exchanges0523201 1a.html

Cromwell, J., Adamache, K. W., Ammering, C., Bartosch, W. J., & Boulis, A. (1995). Equity of the Medicaid Program to the Poor Versus Taxpayers. *Health Care Financing Review*, 75-104.

Definition   of   Externality.   (n.d.).   Retrieved   from   Econterms: http://economics.about.com/cs/economicsglossary/g/externality.htm.

Elmendorf, D. W. (2011, March 30). *CBO's Analysis of the Major Health Care Legislation Enacted in March 2012*. Retrieved July 13, 2012, from CBO: http://www.cbo.gov/sites/default/files/cbofiles/ ftpdocs/121xx/doc12119/03-30-healthcarelegislation.pdf

Emanuel, E. (n.d.). *Here's Why Health Insurance is Not Like Broccoli*. Retrieved July 19, 2012,   from   http://blogs.reuters.com/great-debate/2012/03/29/   heres-why-health-insurance-is-not-like-broccoli/

Essential Health Benefits. (n.d.). Retrieved December 17, 2012, from Cign: http://www.cigna.com/aboutcigna/informed-on-reform/   essential-health-benefits.html

Essential Health Benefits Bulletin. (2011, December 16). Retrieved December 17, 2012, from Center for Consumer Information and Insurance Oversight: http://www.uhc.com/live/uhc_com/Assets/ Documents/Essential_health_benefits_bulletin.pdf

Fernandez, B. (2010, June 7). *Grandfathered Health Plans Under the Patient Protection and Affordable Care Act*. Retrieved July 30, 2012, from National Conference of State Legislators: http://www.ncsl.org/documents/health/Grandfathered Plans.pdf

Foster, R. (2010, April 22). *Estimated Financial Effects of the Patient Protection and Affordable Care Act*. Retrieved August 2, 2012, from CMS.gov: https://www.cms.gov/Research-Statistics-Data-and- Systems/Research/ActuarialStudies/downloads/PPACA_ 2010-04-22.pdf

Fox, D., & Leichter, H. (1991). *Rationing Care in Oregon: The New Accountability*. Retrieved August 12, 2012, from Health Affairs: http://content.healthaffairs.org/content/10/2/7.full.pdf+html?ijkey=1f3dfa96d89 92408f1869b3e4f449f942b34613d&keytype2=tf_ipsecsha

General Accounting Office. (1990). *State and Local Finances: Some Jurisdictions Confronted by Short and Long Term Problems*. Washington, D.C.: General Accounting Office.

Gonzales v. Raich: Implications For Public Health Policy. (2005). *Public Health Representative*, 680-682.

Goodwin, L., & Wilson, C. (2012, June 29). *Map: Where ObamaCare Would Expand Medicaid Most*. Retrieved July 13, 2012, from Yahoo News: http://news.yahoo.com/blogs/ticket/map-where-ObamaCare-expand-medicaid- most-175400889.html

Gordon, D., Long, W., & Killingsworth, P. (2010). *TennCare Oversight Committee Presentation*. Retrieved April 4, 2011, from http:// www.capitol.tn.gov/joint/committees/tenncare/tenncareoversight082410.pdf

Hadley, J., Holahan, J., Coughlin, T., & Miller, D. (2008, August 25). Covering the Unisured in 2008: Current Cost, Sources of Payment, and Incremental Cost. *Health Affairs 27, no. 5*.

Health Connector Commonwealth Care Program Guide. (2012). Retrieved August 19, 2012, from https://www.mahealthconnector.org/portal/binary/com.epicentric. contentmanagement.servlet.ContentDeliveryServlet/About%2520Us/Common wealthCare/Commonwealth%2520Care%2520Program%2520Guide.pdf

Health Insurance 101. (2011). Retrieved December 19, 2012, from Community Catalyst and Georgetown University Health Policy Institute: http://101.communitycatalyst.org/aca_provisions/ subsidies

Health Insurance 101, ACA Provisions. (n.d.). Retrieved December 29, 2012, from CommunityCatalyst: http://101.communitycatalyst.org/aca_provisions/aca_basics

Health Insurance 101, Key Regulation Concepts. (n.d.). Retrieved Decmeber 29, 2012, from http://101.communitycatalyst.org/ key_regulation_concepts?id=0001

Health Insurance 101, Rescissions. (n.d.). Retrieved December 29, 2012, from http://101.communitycatalyst.org/aca_provisions/consumer _protections?id=0004

Health Insurance Explained. (n.d.). Retrieved January 4, 2013, from Insurelane: http://www.insurelane.com/health/health-insurance-explained.html

Health Insurance Reform Enacted State Laws Related to the Affordable Health Care Act. (2011 and 2012). Retrieved July 27, 2012, from National Conference of State

Legislators: http://www.ncsl.org/ issues-research/health/2012-health-insurance-reform-state-laws.aspx

Health Reform in Massachusetts: Expaninding Access to Health Insurance Coverage: Assessing the Results. (2011, April). Retrieved August 17, 2012, from Blue Cross Blue Shield Massachusetts Foundation: http://bluecrossmafoundation.org/ Health-Reform/~/media/D0DDA3D667BE49D58539821 F74C723C7.pdf

Hidden Cost Value Lost, Uninsurance in America. (2003). Retrieved August 10, 2012, from Institute of Medicine (IOM): http://books.nap.edu/openbook.php?record_id=10719&page=R2

Hirschkorn, P., & Glor, J. (2012, June 24). *Massachusetts' Health Care Plan: 6 years Later.* Retrieved August 13, 2012, from CBS News: http://www.cbsnews.com/8301-18563_162-57459563/massachusetts-health-care-plan-6-years-later/

Horsley, S. (2012, August 9). *Doctors Say Health Care Rationing Already Exists.* Retrieved August 9, 2012, from National Public Radio: http://www.npr.org/templates/story/story.php?storyId= 106168331

How Do People Get Health Insurance? (n.d.). Retrieved January 2, 2013, from Health Insurance 101: The Basics: http://101.communitycatalyst.org/basics/overview?id=0002

Hudson, T. (1992). States Scramble for Solutions Under New Medicaid Law. *Hospitals 66, no. 11,* 52-55.

Individual Mandate in Reform. (n.d.). Retrieved December 23, 2012, from Cigna: http://www.cigna.com/aboutcigna/informed-on-reform/individual-mandate.html

Inglehart, J. K. (1994). Health Policy Report: Health Care Reform by the State. *Journal of Medicine 330, no. 1,* 75-79.

Is Health Care Reform Constitutional? (n.d.). Retrieved July 17, 2012, from Constitutionland Development Corporation: http://www.constitution land.com/Health_care_Reform.html

Joyner, J. (2012, March 27). *ObamaCare Mandate Limiting Principle.* Retrieved July 21, 2012, from Outside the Beltway: http://www.outsidethebeltway.com/ObamaCare-mandate-limiting-principle/

Katz, M., & Rosen, H. (1997). *Microeconomics 3rd Edition.* Mcgraw Hill/ Irwin Publishers.

Kennedy, E. M. (2003). Quality, Affordable Health Care for All Americans. *American Journal of Public Health, Volume 93(1),* 14.

Koch, A. (1993). Financing Health Services. In S. J. Williams, & P. R. Torrens, *Introduction to Health Services, 4th Edition* (p. 302). New York, New York: Delmar Publishers Inc.

Ku, L., & Coughlin, T. (1995). Medicaid Disproportionate Share and Other Special Financing Programs. *Health Care Financing Review 16, no. 3,* 1-54.

Kuhn, T. (1970). *The Structure of Scientific Revolutions 3rd ed.* Chicago: The University of Chicago Press.

Leichter, D. F. (1991). Rationing Care in Oregon: The New Accountability. *Health Affairs 10, no. 2,* 7-27.

Local Area Unemployment Statistics: General Overview. (n.d.). Retrieved November 29, 2006, from U.S. Department of Labor, Bureau of Labor Statistics: http://www.bls.gov/lau/home.htm#overview

Lutz, S. (1995). For Real Reform, Watch the States. *Modern Healthcare 25, no. 4,* 30-33.

Mariner, W. (1992). Problems with Employer-Provided Health Insurance: The Employee Retirement Income Security Act and Health Care Reform. *New England Journal of Medicine 327*, 1682-1685.

Massachusetts Health Insurance Requirements. (2012). Retrieved August 14, 2012, from MassResources.org: http://www.mass resources.org/health-reform.html#reformact

MassHealth: General Eligibility Requirements. (2012). Retrieved August 14, 2012, from MassResources.org: http://www.massresources. org/masshealth-general-eligibility.html

Mathews, M. (2012, May 31). *Medicare and Medicaid Fraud Is Costing Taxpayers Billions.* Retrieved July 28, 2012, from Forbes: http://www.forbes.com/sites/merrillmatthews/2012/05/31/medicare-and-medicaid-fraud-is-costing-taxpayers-billions/

McWherter, N. (1993). *TennCare: A New Direction in Health Care.* Nashville: State of Tennessee Report.

Mead, H., Cartwright-Smith, L., Jones, K., Ramos, C., Woods, K., & Siegel, B. (2008). *Racial and Ethnic Disparities in U.S Health Care: A Chart Book, Vol. 27.*

Medicaid. (2012). Retrieved July 14, 2012, from The New York Times: http://topics.nytimes.com/top/news/health/diseasesconditionsandhealthtopics/medicaid/index.html

Medicare Prescription Drug Coverage Part D. (n.d.). Retrieved July 27, 2012, from . http://www.medicare.gov/navigation/medicare-basics/medicare-benefits/part-d.aspx?AspxAutoDetectCookie Support=1#CoverageGap

Medicare Preventive Services. (2012, July 28). Retrieved July 28, 2012, from Healthcare.gov: http://www.healthcare.gov/law/features/ 65-older/medicare-preventive-services/index.html

Mirivis, D. M., Chang, C. F., Hall, C. J., Zaar, G. T., & Applegate, W. B. (1995). TennCare: Health System Reform for Tennessee. *Journal of the American Medical Association 274 no. 15*, 1235.

More States Work to Implement Health Care Law. (2012, May 16). Retrieved July 25, 2012, from U.S. Department of Health and Human Services: http://www.hhs.gov/news/press/2012pres/ 05/2012/20120516a.html

National Federation of Independent Business, et al. v. Sebelius Secretary of Health and Human Services, et al. (2012, June 28). Retrieved July 20, 2012, from http://www.supremecourt.gov/opinions/ 11pdf/11-393c3a2.pdf

New Tools to Fight Fraud, Strengthen Federal and Private Health Programs, and Protect Consumer and Taxpayers Dollars. (2012, July 28). Retrieved July 28, 2012, from Healthcare.gov: http://www.healthcare.gov/news/factsheets/2012/02/medicare-fraud02142012a.html

Nicholson, J. L., Collins, S. R., Mahato, B., Gould, E., Schoen, C., & Rustgi, S. D. (2009). *Rite of Passage? Why Young Adults Become Uninsured and How New Policies Can Help.* Retrieved August 17, 2012, from The CommonWealth Fund Issue Brief: http://www.commonwealthfund.org/~/media/Files/Publications/Issue%20Brief/2009/Aug/1310_Nicholson_rite_of_passage_2009.pdf

Oberlander, J. (2007). *Health Reform Interrupted: The Unraveling of the Oregon Health Plan.* Retrieved August 7, 2010, from Health Affairs: http://content.healthaffairs.org/content/26/1/w96.full

Oregon Health Plan. (n.d.). Retrieved August 8, 2012, from Oregon.gov: http://cms.oregon.gov/oha/healthplan/pages/priorlist/main.aspx

Oregon   Live.   (2011,   April   7).   Retrieved   August   13,   2012,   from
        http://www.oregonlive.com/health/index.ssf/2011/04/gov_john_kitzhaber_want
        s_to_gi.html

Palmer, K. S. (1999). *A Brief History: Universal Care Efforts in the US.* Retrieved
        August 19, 2012, from Physicians for a National Health Program:
        http://www.pnhp.org/facts/a-brief-history-universal-health-care-efforts-in-the-
        us

Preventive Services. (n.d.). Retrieved July 28, 2012, from Medicare.gov:
        http://www.medicare.gov/navigation/manage-your-health/   preventive-
        services/preventive-service-overview.aspx

Reinhardt, U. (2009, July 3). *Rationing, Health Care: What Does it Mean?* Retrieved
        August   10,   2012,   from   New   York   Times:
        http://economix.blogs.nytimes.com/2009/07/03/rationing-health-care-what-
        does-it-mean/

Remarks by the President on Supreme Court Ruling on the Affordable Care Act. (2012,
        June   28).   Retrieved   July   14,   2012,   from   The   White   House:
        http://www.whitehouse.gov/the-press-office/2012/   06/28/remarks-president-
        supreme-court-ruling-affordable-care-act

Roemer, M. I. (1978). *Social Medicine: The Advance of Organized health Services in
        America.* New York: Springer.

Rognehaugh, R. (1998). *The Managed Health Care Dictionary 2nd ed.* Gaithersburg,
        Maryland: Aspen Publishers, Inc.

Roy, A. (2012, July 24). *CBO Guesstimates that the Supreme Court's Impact on
        ObamaCare   is   Modest.*   Retrieved   August   3,   2012,   from   Forbes:
        http://www.forbes.com/sites/aroy/2012/07/24/cbo-guesstimates-that-
        ObamaCare-will-cover-3-million-less-people-after-the-supreme-court-saving-
        84-billion/

Schoen, C., Osborn, R., How, S. K., Doty, M. M., & Peugh, J. (2008). *In Chronic
        Conditions: Experiences of Patients With Complex Health Care Needs in Eight
        Countries.*   Retrieved   2012,   from   Health   Affairs:
        http://content.healthaffairs.org/content/28/1/w1.full.pdf+html?sid=274e8699-
        1920-4065-a257-1ff2ea0d80f3

Smith, S., Freeland, M., Heffler, S., McKusick, D., & Health Expenditures Projection
        Team. (1998). The Next Ten Years of Health Spending: What Does the Future
        Hold? *Health Affairs 17, no. 5,* 128-140.

Social Security Bulletin 83. (1994). Washington, D.C.: U.S. Department of Health and
        Human Services.

Social Security Programs in the United States, Bulletin 56, no. 4. (1993). Washington,
        D.C.: U.S. Department of Health and Human Services.

State by State Enrollment in the Preexisting Insurance Plan. (2012, April 30).   Retrieved
        July 26, 2012, from HealthCare.gov: http://www.healthcare.gov/news/fact
        sheets/2012/06/pcip06152012a.html

Stevens, R. (2007, September 21). *History & Health Policy in the United States: Putting
        the Past Back.* Retrieved August 7, 2012, from Investigator Awards:
        http://www.investigatorawards.org/downloads/research_in_
        profiles_iss21_sep2007.pdf

Summary of Benefits and Coverage. (n.d.). Retrieved December 29, 2012, from Cigna:
        http://www.cigna.com/aboutcigna/informed-on-reform/   summary-of-benefits-
        and-coverage.html

Take Charge of Your Health. (n.d.). Retrieved September 3, 2012, from Aetna: http://healthinsurance.aetna.com/media/pdf_plans/TN_ Direct.pdf

TennCare Information. (2006). Retrieved December 15, 2010, from THA: http://www.tha.com/pdffiles/THA-Legisl-Conf-2006/2006-TennCare-Reform.pdf

The Hawaii Prepaid Health Care Act. (n.d.). *State of Hawaii*, pp. Section 393: 1-53.

Timeline of Provisions. (n.d.). Retrieved December 16, 2012, from UnitedHealthcare: http://www.uhc.com/united_for_reform_   resource_ center/health_reform_provisions/essential_health_benefits.htm

Torrens, P. R. (1993). Historical Evolution of Health Services in the United States. In S. J. Williams, & P. R. Torrens, *Introduction to Health Services, 4th Edition* (pp. 14-28). New York, New York: Delmar Publishers Inc.

Understanding Aetna. (n.d.). Retrieved Septemeber 3, 2012, from Aetna.com: http://www.aetna.com/plans-services-health-insurance/detail/assets/documents/Member-brochure.pdf

United States v. Comstock et al. (2010, May 17). Retrieved July 22, 2012, from http://www.supremecourt.gov/opinions/09pdf/08-1224.pdf

Updated Estimates for the Insurance Coverage Provisions of the Affordable   Care Act. (2012, March). Retrieved January 10, 2013, from Congressional Budget Office: http://www.cbo.gov/sites/   default/files/cbofiles/attachments/03-13-Coverage%20Estimates.pdf

U.S. Supreme Court and the Federal Health Law. (2012, July 24). Retrieved August 5, 2012, from National Conference of State Legislators (NCSL): http://www.ncsl.org/issues-research/ health/us-supreme-court-and-the-federal-health-law.aspx

Watson, S. D. (1995). Medicaid Physicin Participation: Patients, Poverty, and Physician Self Interest. *American Journal of Law and Medicine no. 42*, 142-151.

What is Medicare? (n.d.). Retrieved July 26, 2012, from Centers for Medicare and Medicaid Services: http://www.medicare.gov/ publications/pubs/pdf/11306.pdf

Why Do You Need Health Insurance? (n.d.). Retrieved Januray 7, 2013, from Agency For Health   Care   Reasearch   and   Quality: http:// archive.ahrq.gov/consumer/insuranceqa/insuranceqa3.htm

Your Medicare Coverage Choices. (n.d.). Retrieved June 29, 2012, from Medicare.gov: http://www.medicare.gov/navigation/medicare-basics/coverage-choices.aspx

Index

About the Author

Chinyere Chigozie Ogbonna was born in Okwe, Nigeria. She completed her elementary education at Ekulu Primary School, Enugu in 1980. She graduated from Federal Government College, Enugu in 1985. She earned a Bachelor of Science Degree (Honors) in Parasitology and Entomology from Anambara State University, Enugu, Nigeria in 1990 and a Master of Science Degree in Health Care Administration from Western Kentucky University in 1996. Her Doctorate in Public Administration was earned at Tennessee State University in August 2000.

Dr. Ogbonna has held various positions in both private and public health care industries, including research positions at Vanderbilt and Vectors /Arbovirus Research division under the auspices of World Health Organization and in 2001 she served as Bioterrorism Epidemiologist for Tennessee Department of Health. She worked in Administration at the office of International programs at Western Kentucky University. She is the author of TennCare and Disproportionate Share Hospitals and the main author of the 2009 book, Voices from the Inside. Dr. Ogbonna is currently employed as an Associate Professor of Public Management and Criminal Justice at Austin Peay State University, Clarksville, Tennessee.